WAY

D0622787

**ALLEN COUNTY PUBLIC LIBRARY
FORT WAYNE, INDIANA 46802**

You may return this book to any agency, branch,
or bookmobile of the Allen County Public Library

DEMCO

DISCOVER
OSTEOPATHY

FUNDS TO PURCHASE
THIS BOOK WERE
PROVIDED BY A
40TH ANNIVERSARY GRANT
FROM THE
FOELLINGER FOUNDATION.

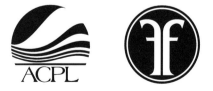

DISCOVER OSTEOPATHY

PETA SNEDDON AND PAOLO COSESCHI

KATHERINE ARMITAGE
Illustrator

Ulysses Press 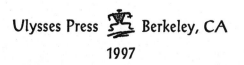 Berkeley, CA

1997

This book has been written and published strictly for informational purposes, and in no way should it be used as a substitute for consultation with your medical doctor or other health care professional. All facts in this book came from medical files, clinical journals, scientific publications, personal interviews, published trade books, self-published materials by experts, magazine articles, and the personal-practice experiences of the authorities quoted or sources cited. You should not consider educational material herein to be the practice of medicine or to replace consultation with a physician or other medical practitioner. The author and publisher are providing you with information in this work so that you can have the knowledge and can choose, at your own risk, to act on that knowledge. The author and publisher also urge all readers to be aware of their health status and to consult health professionals before beginning any health program, including changes in dietary habits.

All names and identifying characteristics of real persons have been changed in the text to protect their confidentiality.

Published by: Ulysses Press
         P.O. Box 3440
         Berkeley, CA 94703-3440

Library of Congress Catalog Card Number: 97-60158

ISBN: 1-56975-115-3

Printed in the USA by the George Banta Company

First published as *Healing With Osteopathy*, Gill & Macmillan, 1996

10 9 8 7 6 5 4 3 2 1

Editorial and production: Leslie Henriques, Claire Chun, Lily Chou, Nicole O'Hay
Typesetter: David Wells
Cover Design: B & L Design
Indexer: Sayre Van Young

Distributed in the United States by Publishers Group West and in Canada by Raincoast Books

TABLE OF CONTENTS

ACKNOWLEDGMENTS

We would like to thank the following: Marian Faulkner, who has spent many hours going through the manuscript with us, and without whom this book would not have taken its shape; Patrizia Lacerna and Danile degli Angeli for their advice and suggestions; our patients, who make our learning an ongoing process; all our teachers, particularly Thomas Dummer, Harold Klug, Susan Turner and Gerald Lamb, who are a source of constant inspiration.

PART ONE

—

THE ORIGINS AND BASICS OF OSTEOPATHY

THE HISTORY OF OSTEOPATHY

———

The dawning of Western medicine as we know it today began at the time of the Greek civilization in the fourth century B.C., when two main schools of thought started guiding and shaping medicine. One school was founded by Hippocrates, who emphasized that the whole individual as a unique being needed to be studied and treated for good health. The second school was founded in the town of Knidos, its followers concentrating on looking at disease as an invader that had to be destroyed — medical intervention was aimed at directly relieving the symptoms of disease.

Throughout the history of medicine these two conflicting approaches can be traced, and the split can still be found in modern orthodox medical treatment. While the medical profession has always recognized its origin in Hippocratic thought, conventional medical treatment uses the Knidian approach in attacking and trying to eradicate disease.

Over the centuries, though, there have been various people in medicine who have reaffirmed the Hippocratic approach. In the seventeenth century, the father of modern clinical methods, Dr. T. Sydenham, brought his students back to the patient's bedside, showing them that only there could they learn about disease.

Dr. Andrew Still, the founder of osteopathy, believed that a healing process should involve the whole person, and that every local problem had to be treated in the context of the whole being. Dr. Still stressed that in order to promote a more profound healing, it was necessary to trace and treat the mechanical imbalance that lies behind the disease process.

ANDREW TAYLOR STILL

The founder of osteopathy was born in 1828, the son of a Methodist camp-fire preacher/country doctor Abram Still and his wife Martha. At the age of nine, Andrew Still moved with his family to Macon County, Missouri, where the frontier life he led formed the basis of his understanding of the "great book of nature," even before his study of anatomy.

In 1852, Andrew Still went to live with part of his family in Indian County, Kansas. There he spent the next twenty-one years, and began what he called the science of osteopathy. From his father he received his first medical training, and his evangelical character. Branching out on his own years later, he also left all forms of organized religion.

Dr. Still developed his theory and healing methods at a particularly dark moment in the medical history of the U.S. His experiences as an army doctor during the Civil War in 1861 deeply shook his trust in the medicine of the time. The devastation brought about by infected wounds, infections following operations, the uselessness of most medicines, and the epidemics that followed the end of the war were very traumatic for him. In addition, three of his children and his young wife died during a spinal meningitis epidemic.

He turned to the study of man, paying attention to what good health is rather than concentrating on disease. With the conviction that God must have put within man's nature the means for self-healing, he began an in-depth study of human anatomy.

FORMATIVE INFLUENCES

As he began to move away from conventional medical practices, Still was greatly influenced by two men. The first was J. B. Abbott, a scholar who told Still that a new discipline would emerge to take the place of orthodox forms of medicine of the time. Dr. Still then became interested in phrenology, mesmerism, spiritualism and magnetic healing (see the Glossary for definitions of all these practices).

The second and even greater influence on Still was the philosopher Herbert Spencer. In his book *First Principles*, Spencer was the one who first used the term evolution. Still borrowed from Spencer and then elaborated on such osteopathic concepts as cause and effect, structure and function, and the holistic working of the body. Later, Still pointed out in his work the importance of mind-matter-motion as the basis of osteopathic principles. For Still, "mind" was the life within all living things.

MAGNETIC HEALING

Some time after moving to Missouri in the 1870s, Still opened his first office, as a magnetic healer. Practitioners of magnetic healing believed that an invisible fluid — animal magnetism — flowed through the body, which when in balance meant good health for the individual (see the Glossary). From 1883, he began to introduce bone-setting procedures in his treatment, while developing his thinking, which was based on evolutionary principles and research on the nervous system. This led him to establish a scientific basis for his manipulative techniques, and he then abandoned magnetic healing. Still may be thought of as having taken the old art of bone-setting and turned and developed it into a proper system of medicine.

THE AMERICAN SCHOOL OF OSTEOPATHY (ASO)

As his practice grew steadily, Still opened the ASO in 1892, with eleven students. At the school, Still taught his students that disease could result from strains, shocks and other traumas that could alter the blood circulation and the activity of the body's nervous system.

Practitioners of alternative methods of healing in the U.S. were seen as a threat by the medical profession, yet osteopathy and indeed homeopathy continued to grow in popularity. A number of osteopathic schools were established in the 1890s. Still then became aware of the struggle to keep osteopathy pure, as some students wished to use drugs as well as osteopathic techniques in treating patients.

Eventually, the training of osteopaths in the U.S. was to merge with the training of orthodox medical physicians.

NEW DEVELOPMENTS

Andrew Still died in 1917, having left behind him a legacy of enormous importance to the healing therapies. From his teaching, such osteopathic practitioners as William Garner Sutherland flourished going on to build further on Still's theories and practices. Sutherland's studies led him to believe that a movement existed in the cranium (the skull), a movement called the primary respiratory mechanism (see Chapter Six).

John Martin Littlejohn, a Scotsman who studied with Still, enlarged the focus of osteopathy by concentrating not only on the anatomy but stressing the physiological aspect. Contrary to Still, Littlejohn wanted osteopaths to learn all about modern medicine as well as osteopathic principles and practices. Eventually, Littlejohn returned to Britain, where he founded the British School of Osteopathy.

OSTEOPATHY IN THE U.S.

There are some 38,000 osteopathic physicians and surgeons in the U.S. They have the letters DO (Doctor of Osteopathic Medicine) after their name, and they have the same rights to practice as MDs (Medical Doctors) in every state in the country. Most of them choose to be primary care physicians, although few of them work only with their hands.

In 1967, there were six colleges of osteopathic medicine in the U.S. Due to the rapid growth of the profession in the 1970s, there are now seventeen such colleges.

Although osteopathic medicine represents only five per cent of the physician population in the U.S., it is a fast-growing part of the health-care field. Osteopathic physicians work and study side by side with orthodox physicians in many health-care settings. At the same time, the profession is maintaining its independence and developing and perpetuating its unique system of medicine.

THE FUTURE

In the 120 years since Dr. Still founded osteopathy, the profession he began has become a world-wide discipline. Osteopathy has achieved statutory recognition, and is a part of the health-care system in almost all of the English-speaking countries and in many others.

In the 1990s, we can see the rise of a new, more global approach to human health. This is coming about because of more research and increased communication between the different therapies in medicine. Working together is the key note for a new development in the medical arts. *Discover Osteopathy* has arisen out of the hope that this collaboration will flourish, and out of the source of inspiration that the discipline of osteopathy has been in our own lives. As this book forms an introduction to the complex subject of osteopathy, we have been selective about the specialist areas in which osteopathy may be applied. We regret that it has not been possible to cover more!

2

WHAT IS OSTEOPATHY?

———

Osteopathy is a distinctive and complete system of health care, based on broad principles that "offer a way of thinking and acting in relation to questions of health and disease" (Dr. I. M. Korr). The procedures it uses in diagnosis and treatment promote healthy functioning in a person by correcting mechanical imbalances within and between the structures of the body. By structures we mean the muscles, bones, ligaments, organs and fascia. The fascia is a very thin layer of tissue that is found under the skin (see the Glossary). Correcting the mechanical imbalances in the structures is done by restoring, maintaining and improving the harmonious working of the nervous and musculoskeletal systems.

The name osteopathy (given to the therapy by Dr. Still) comes from the Greek *osteon* (bone) and *pathos* (to suffer), so it literally means suffering of the bone. The name has created some confusion, leading people to think that an osteopath treats only conditions of the bones. However, Dr. Still chose the name because he recognized the importance of a properly functioning musculoskeletal system for the total well-being of the individual.

HUMAN ANATOMY

The greatest interest of practitioners of osteopathy is the study of human anatomy and physiology. Following in Dr. Still's footsteps, they know how important it is to have a thorough understanding of the correct position and function of each bone and other structures in the body. This is essential in order to find out about the normal and healthy working of the human body. Those working in osteopathy look at the causes of disease and suffering originating in the abnormal working relationship that can exist within and between structures.

Dr. Still thought of the musculoskeletal system as the primary machinery of life and saw how disruptions in this delicate machine may lead to illness. For the osteopath, therefore, the physical integrity of the whole body is seen as one of the most important factors in health and disease. Rather than bone specialists, osteopaths are in fact masters in the biomechanics of the human machine.

OSTEOPATHY AND MEDICINE

Osteopathy and orthodox medicine have many things in common: they both use the scientific knowledge of anatomy and physiology, as well as clinical methods of investigation. In this respect, they have a similar language. The greatest differences, however, lie in the way patients are evaluated and in the approach to treatment.

As a general rule, the orthodox medical approach focuses on the end product of the problem — that is, on the illness. This

The Vertebral Column

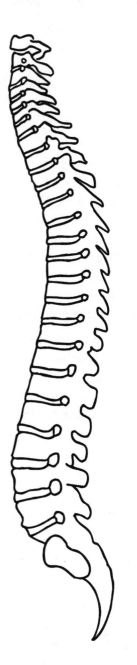

Cervical spine, composed of
7 vertebrae, from C1 to C7

Dorsal spine, composed of
12 vertebrae, from D1 to D12

Lumbar spine, composed of
5 vertebrae, from L1 to L5

Sacrum, composed of
5 fused vertebrae

follows from finding the pathogen, chemical disturbance or structural pathology (for all these terms, see the Glossary). Treatment aims to redress the balance by giving drugs or carrying out surgery.

Osteopaths focus on tracing the changes in function that have occurred over a period of time. This is in order to try to understand the chain of events that have altered the relationship between structure and function, resulting in the present complaint.

A typical example might be a six-year-old boy who, while playing, falls very hard on his bottom. He cries bitterly and complains of pain over his sacrum (see the Glossary) for a week or so. A kiss and "rub it better" console him. During a sudden growth spurt as a teenager, the same boy complains of low back ache. By the age of eighteen, he has his first attack of sciatica, which is helped by anti-inflammatory and muscle relaxant medicine. He gives up his favorite sport, rowing, because it seems to aggravate the problem.

In his late twenties, married with a young child and a stressful job, he begins to have an irritable colon and attacks of cystitis. He takes antibiotics and changes his diet. At the age of forty he has a major attack of low back pain and sciatica and is in bed for two weeks. At this point, hoping to avoid surgery, he visits an osteopath.

HOMEOSTASIS AND THE SYSTEMS THEORY

The belief in the self-healing capacity of the body is very ancient, and in our Western medical tradition it can be traced back to Hippocrates. Dr. Still reaffirmed this belief at a time when it was particularly needed, and before the discovery of the law of homeostasis.

Homeostasis is the process by which every living thing makes continual adjustments to keep itself in a stable condition and function to the best of its ability. It is a self-regulating activity, with pre-set limits. For example, in the blood there must be a precise quantity of dissolved oxygen within maximum and minimum levels in order for all the body tissues to work. The body is constantly readjusting to maintain this balance.

The in-built homeostatic mechanism comes into play to restore balance where it has been disrupted and it is the result of the biological cognitive (see the Glossary) process. This occurs in every cell in the body, involving a kind of memory that is not limited to our brain and conscious thought. In this sense, the whole of our physical structure is but a bank of memories.

THE LIVING SYSTEM

Modern biology and cognitive science (the study of how we know what we know) can give us a better insight into some of Dr. Still's theories and beliefs. Every living thing, from a single cell to the earth itself, can be seen as a living system. To see how the principles of osteopathy are rooted in our physiological make up, we can take the example of one individual cell.

When in the presence of an irritant, the cell changes its wall to protect itself, and stabilizes its internal network of communications. The result is that the life within the cell is kept in balance, through its self-adjusting, "thinking" responses. The ability to do this is found in each cell throughout the body. A cell, like any other living system, is considered to be both closed and open. It is closed because it always refers to its internal organization in its exchanges with the world around it. It is able to construct its own inner environment and is self-generating. A cell is an open system because it is able to modify its structure in response to the stimuli it receives from outside. A living system is therefore open because it is influenced by and responds to its outside environment. This leads us on to another important aspect of a living organism, which is the tendency to self-improvement.

Systems theory shows the depth of the structure-function relationship that is found in each and every cell of the body. This is not limited to the cell, but involves the functioning of the whole of the physical body as well as giving us an insight into the way we relate both to ourselves and to the external world. By affirming the existence of a "total body memory" and our inherent capacity for balance and self-improvement, we can understand how the self-healing power of the body is often helped by the *minimum* of therapeutic intervention. Clearly, this theory also supports and justifies an holistic approach to health.

THE SELF-HEALING MECHANISM

Osteopaths believe that health, and not disease, is the natural heritage of man. The human body has inside itself — within certain limits — the capacity for self-repair and correction. It can create its own remedies, provided that good circulation is maintained, a balanced diet is eaten, a positive attitude is held and — as far as possible — you live in a pollution-free environment.

The self-healing mechanism is the backbone and sustainer of the principles and application of osteopathy. Osteopaths believe that disease primarily comes from within the individual, and so they concentrate on the person who is suffering rather than on the microorganisms that are thought to cause disease. There are, however, some stages of disease where the changes it has brought about have gone beyond the point of return. In these cases, osteopathy can help the person to function to the best of his ability, given the circumstances. Where necessary, an osteopath will refer a patient for further specialist examination and treatment.

THE PRINCIPLES OF OSTEOPATHY

Three of the main principles of osteopathy are:

1. Structure and function are interdependent

2. "The rule of the artery is supreme"

3. The unity of the human being

1. STRUCTURE AND FUNCTION ARE INTERDEPENDENT

Life is a dynamic process in which change is the only constant and so its main characteristic is motion. Motion — or movement — within a healthy, balanced body (or any other living thing) is fluid and rhythmical. Free movement between the body structures is essential for the health of an individual. When it is disrupted the function is in some way disturbed. Disrupted movement is the altered state that comes about before disease emerges.

When we use the term structure, we mean the muscles, bones ligaments, organs and fascia (see the Glossary). By the term function, we mean the way in which all the different parts of the body work within themselves and in relation to each other. The relationship between structure and function applied in a therapeutic context is probably the greatest contribution made by Andrew Still to medicine. A very good example of this relationship is the young, growing brain. The amount of varied activity that stimulates the brain to work also influences the rate and quality of the growth of the brain tissue itself.

The structure of the circulatory system is the heart, blood vessels, their valves and the blood. If the blood vessel walls get thicker and harder — which may be caused by an imbalance in the contents of the blood — then problems may develop in the circulation.

The osteopath looks for free movement between the joints. In the spine, for example, she looks for flexibility and mobility, as without these the blood and nerve supply to the surrounding and related tissues and organs will be poor. In treatment, the osteopath aims to have a positive effect on the body's function, even though she works directly on the structure.

2. "THE RULE OF THE ARTERY IS SUPREME"

This expression means that, for good health, good circulation of all body fluids is essential. Poor circulation is likely to mean that the cells will be starved of what they need to survive, and will eventually die. All the tissues in the body are made up of different kinds of cells, which get their nutrients from the fluid in which they live. The body fluid consists of the blood, lymph, which drains and cleans the tissues, and the spinal fluid that supports, nourishes and drains the central nervous system. In order for the nutrients to be easily absorbed and for waste products to be got rid of, three conditions need to be fulfilled:

• the fluid must be present in sufficient quantity

• the rhythmic movement of the cells must be constant

• the body fluids must circulate freely

The circulatory system carries the hormones produced by the endocrine system and is controlled by the nervous system. The two systems that form a communication between all the systems of the body are the nervous and circulatory systems. In his writing, Dr. Still often emphasized the importance of one particular system — the musculoskeletal system, the lymphatic system, the fascia, etc. The reason for this was probably his intuition that in each individual case, one system was the most important factor in creating the disease. At the same time, he always maintained his vision of the unity of the whole body.

3. THE UNITY OF THE HUMAN BEING

According to the Western Christian tradition, the human being consists of a threefold unit: body, mind and spirit. This view was adopted by many of the first osteopaths and it is still held by many practitioners today. The relationship between the mind and the body is now taken into consideration by most physicians and health-care professionals. The effect of emotions such as fear, laughter or sadness on the body, for example, is immediately apparent.

This unity of the body and its self-healing capacity is also evident in the neurological, endocrine and immune systems. In the past decade, researchers have discovered that chemical substances (a variety of hormones and neurological transmitters) produced by the body are recognized by and communicate with these three systems. This process is a means by which the body sets in motion its healing mechanism.

For example, an inflammation in the tissues results in the release of substances that increase circulation and temperature and cause increased sensitivity or even pain by irritating the nerve endings. This information travels in the spinal cord, and some of it goes to the brain, where it stimulates the release of hormones into the blood. It also brings to our conscious awareness the local problem. Once in circulation around the body, these hormones will affect different organs and interact with the immune system. In this way, the whole body is woken up and works as a complete unit to bring things back to normal.

The nervous and circulatory systems not only integrate the normal functions of the body but, if disturbed, can inhibit the body's natural powers of self-healing. The body's musculoskeletal system reflects, and may aggravate, the condition of these systems and so influence a person's state of health. When an osteopath thinks of the interconnectedness of the body he has in his mind all of these systems.

OSTEOPATHY AND THE HOLISTIC APPROACH

A holistic approach to health means that every part of the body is seen within the context of the whole; that whole is *more* than the sum of the parts. As all the organs and systems of the body are interconnected, we cannot treat one part without influencing and changing the whole. This may mean that the cause of a problem may be far from where the symptoms are found.

A patient who has had a whiplash injury in a car accident, for example, may complain of pain in the leg. Tension in the lower back may be causing this pain, but as the primary problem is located in the neck, until this is resolved there is little chance that the symptoms will clear. The osteopath will therefore take great care in treating the neck as well as the leg and back. This approach will release the stress in the nervous system and help the body to recover as a whole.

PRACTICING OSTEOPATHY

Dr. Andrew Still said: "Find it, fix it and leave it alone." These words sum up how the principles of osteopathy may be applied to treatment. As the path to cure lies inside the patient's body, treatment is directed toward removing some of the obstacles that are stopping the healing process from taking place spontaneously. Overtreatment is a mistake — the osteopath must respect each patient's own rhythms and the pace at which each person functions and so can heal. The practitioner needs to offer the space and time for the individual to carry out their own self-healing.

By acknowledging the uniqueness of each individual, in every treatment session there is a key point for the mind and body which, if properly corrected, will in time bring about a broad and deep change in that person's situation. In order to find the key point, the osteopath must be, as much as possible, in tune with the patient.

What is Healing?

Dr. Still emphasized in all his books the importance of mind-matter-motion. He identified "mind" with man's spiritual being, which can maintain the body in good health only by tuning in to nature's "mind." Behind this, for Still, lay the will of God, the Mind of all minds. Motion was central to Still's thinking because he saw in it the very expression of life.

With this as a starting point, we can say that health is a dynamic process characterized by every aspect of a human being — the thinking, social, physical and spiritual components that go to make up the whole person. A deep healing cannot take place without the combination of all of these parts in our lives.

The way in which the body and mind are linked in the process of healing may be as follows. Within ourselves, we have a series of built-in, automatic reflexes ranging from the physiological homeostatic mechanisms we have looked at above to those that regulate our behavior patterns. These mechanisms can become locked in a circle of self-repetition that may eventually lead to disease. An example of this may be a person who has been under a great deal of stress; because of this he develops an increasing level of anxiety and starts to eat compulsively. This in turn may in time lead to diabetes. So a conditioned pattern of behavior becomes locked in a vicious, self-repeating circle.

Another example could be an elderly woman who breaks her hip. Consequently she is bedridden for several weeks, becomes depressed, loses interest in food and eventually dies prematurely.

On the other hand, we also have a natural tendency toward self-improvement, which means that we can function more efficiently both psychologically and physically. Psychologically, this tendency is characterized by the conscious effort we make toward an increasing self-awareness that can break down unbalanced, conditioned behavior and be our source of continual growth.

Healing spans an extremely wide range, from getting rid of a common cold to achieving a well-balanced personality. It is of course not necessary to go through a deep inner change in order to cure a cold. On the other hand, to heal from serious illness such as cancer may require — along with the appropriate medication — a total transformation and an awakening. Healing goes hand in hand with a feeling of well-being and the return to a joyous personality.

TREATMENT AND HEALING

Healing does not always coincide with treatment. Whether the treatment takes the form of manual manipulation, surgery, drugs or counseling, healing will not always follow and may come about months or years after clinical treatment. One definition of healing may therefore be that a person is functioning to the best of her potential and is therefore healthy. An example of this is a child who, after a fracture, has one leg slightly shorter than the other. He suffers from low back pain and has a limp; he may also have problems with his digestion and difficulty in sleeping. Osteopathic treatment may help with the back pain, digestive and sleeping problems, but the length of the child's leg may be irreparable. So we could say that he is healing when he is back to functioning as well as he can, given that circumstance.

OSTEOPATHY AND OTHER THERAPIES

CHIROPRACTIC

Chiropractic and osteopathy both had their origins in the U.S. toward the end of the nineteenth century. Dr. Daniel Palmer, the founder of chiropractic, is believed to have spent some time studying with Dr. Still. Following that study, Dr. Palmer moved to another state and started his own personal healing discipline. Chiropractic means manual treatment — it is formed by two Greek words, *chiro*, meaning hands, and *praktikos*, meaning done by.

There are similarities and differences between the two therapies. Palmer first stressed the role of the nervous system and of the spinal column in health and disease, seeing nerve compression as the basis for all problems. Chiropractors are more likely to use X-rays when diagnosing a patient's problem. They also concentrate on manipulation of the spine, directly adjusting it with rapid movements. (See the Glossary.)

PHYSIOTHERAPY

The differences between osteopathy and physiotherapy are mainly found in their underlying philosophies. They do not use drugs, but manual treatment, exercises and electrotherapies. In the past, physiotherapists did not make diagnoses, but worked with a patient after the doctor's diagnosis.

Physiotherapists are experts in their field and they work in collaboration with osteopaths in various cases. Over the past hundred years of its life, the profession has changed greatly and it is interesting to see how the attitude and approach of physiotherapists has come to appreciate other methods of treatment. They maintain that they are moving toward a more holistic approach to health and patient management.

3

THE OSTEOPATHIC LESION

—

WHAT IS AN OSTEOPATHIC LESION?

The terms osteopathic lesion and somatic dysfunction are synonymous: they describe what an osteopath looks for in an area of the body where there is a problem. The word lesion in osteopathy has a different meaning from the one it has for an orthodox medical doctor, where it refers to tissue damage due to injury or disease. So in osteopathy, fractures, inflammations and degenerative problems — for example, rheumatoid arthritis — are not thought of as lesions. Osteopathic lesions are functional disturbances that in the long term may play a role in the process of a serious organic illness.

We can see this more clearly by looking at the example of rheumatoid arthritis. It is a degenerative, auto-immune inflammatory disease, involving more than one system (the musculoskeletal, respiratory, circulatory, etc.). The bony joints degenerate, becoming swollen and deformed. An osteopathic lesion in these circumstances could be both muscle contracture, which makes the joint stiffness and pain worse, and central nervous system compression, reflected in a reduced movement of the primary respiratory mechanism (see Chapter Six). This, indirectly, will deplete the body's vitality, reducing its capacity to combat the inflammation.

Osteopathic lesions are created by the mechanical and physiological reaction in the body to various types of trauma. By the expression mechanical, we mean the relationship between body structures. Physiological means the way in which the body works. When speaking of the physiological movement, or motion, of the spine or vertebral column, we are referring to its free, natural movement. By trauma we mean not only physical trauma such as a fall, but also following an operation or an infection, or a difficult birth, emotional trauma, etc.

In osteopathy, free balanced movement is the most important factor in health; the lack of it plays a major part in disease. So all the different techniques used by an osteopath are concerned with re-establishing normal mobility and motility (see the Glossary). To summarize, the osteopathic lesion is a functional disturbance in the body, involving muscles, joints, fascia, the organs and the related parts of the circulatory and nervous systems. Osteopaths, therefore, look for the disturbance in the relationships between these different systems.

WHERE AND HOW DO LESIONS OCCUR?

Somatic dysfunction may occur primarily in any structure of the body, although those involving the spine, or vertebral column, are of special importance. The vertebral column joins the head to the pelvis; the spinal cord, which is part of the central nervous system, passes through the center of it. All the nerves that control the muscles and connect to the internal organs branch out from the spinal cord.

When a vertebra is held in an abnormal or restricted range of movement, the osteopath can see this abnormality as well as feel its restricted mobility. The nervous system "holds" the vertebra in this position by sending abnormal nerve impulses to the muscles and ligaments attached to the vertebra. This may be a local problem in the nervous system, which can cause changes in the texture and quality of the skin, muscles, fascia, ligaments and tendons, which the osteopath will look for.

When we refer to an osteopathic lesion of the spinal joint, we do not speak of "bones being out of place," but of the joint being held in a restricted arc of movement. For example, if the muscles in the neck are tighter on the right, the vertebrae will turn more easily to the right where the muscles are shortened and contracted. On the other hand, turning to the left will be more difficult.

Any osteopathic lesion is recognizable through touch, using a method called palpation (see the Glossary). In a severe lesion that has occurred only recently, the skin feels warm, perhaps sweaty and swollen, due to a build-up of fluid in the tissues under the surface. The muscles will be tense and tender to touch, while the skin may be red in color and more sensitive than normal. If the condition has been present for some time, the skin will feel cooler, drier and thicker; the muscles will feel tense and stringy; the patient may complain of stiffness in the joint.

THE NERVOUS SYSTEM

In order to understand what is meant by osteopathic lesion and facilitation, which plays an important role in it (see the Glossary), you need first of all to have a basic understanding of the nervous system.

In the Western medical model, the nervous system is divided into the following subcategories:

- the central nervous system (brain and spinal cord)
- the peripheral nervous system (the nerves supplying the body).

The nervous system is also sub-categorized as follows:

- somatic nervous system
- autonomic nervous system (see the Glossary).

The somatic nervous system is that part of the system that responds to conscious will. Motor, or efferent, nerves instruct the body to act, while afferent nerves bring messages in for the body to interpret and act upon.

The autonomic nervous system is physically distinct from the somatic nervous system. Ordinarily, the autonomic nervous system works without the influence of the mind to regulate the body — that is, it functions involuntarily. This system is subdivided into the:

- sympathetic nervous system
- parasympathetic nervous system.

The sympathetic nervous system is what prompts us to be "switched on" and act in response to a given situation, either external or internal. The parasympathetic nervous system prompts us to slow down for rest and recovery. When the sympathetic nervous system is activated, our muscles tighten, our breath quickens, our eyes dilate; in extreme cases, the hairs on the body rise, the digestion slows and circulatory changes are brought about. Our attention is turned outward as we assess our situation. In this state, the rest that the body needs in order to recharge its batteries is deferred.

By contrast, when the parasympathetic nervous system is activated, our attention turns inward. The muscles relax, the breath becomes slower and deeper and feelings of tension are replaced by feelings of peace and calm.

The sympathetic and parasympathetic nervous systems complement each other and need to work in harmony for a person to be in balance. This balance cannot be achieved simply by the activity of the somatic nervous system — that is, by an act of will. However, it has been observed that emotional states such as anxiety, which is linked with excessive activity of the sympathetic nervous system and an increased rate of breathing, can be calmed down by an adjustment in the way we breathe.

The different parts of the nervous system are intimately related, both structurally and functionally. All of the nerve fibers in the body are formed by neurons (see the Glossary). The voluntary and involuntary parts of the nervous system communicate with each other via the interneuron, which is found inside the spinal cord. Information can pass to and from the systems and the brain, making the spread of nerve impulses possible and creating a chain of reflexes.

FACILITATION

Abnormal reflexes and facilitation together form most of the different kinds of osteopathic lesions. Let us now look more closely at what facilitation is. Muscles and tendons are full of nerve endings which measure the range and rate of muscle lengthening and shortening. These nerve endings constantly send information back to the central nervous system.

We can compare the driver of a car with the central nervous system, with the car as the body. For example, a driver going at a normal speed sees a child crossing the road in front of him. He has to break, which he can do without damage to himself or his car because the situation is under his control. If our driver's car is instead suddenly hit from behind by another speeding car, he cannot control the situation and his car will be badly damaged.

In such a situation, the central nervous system (the driver) has to face unexpected stress, and reacts by suddenly contracting the relevant muscles. This is done to protect the body from moving beyond its preset limits and damaging itself badly. At this point, the central nervous system and the muscles are on alert; the disturbance in the nerves keeps the muscles contracted, and the other way around.

Even when the driver feels he has recovered from the shock of the accident, there may still be some nerve fibers which keep repeating to each other "Danger! Watch out! Don't let go!" In this way, a vicious circle is created, which holds the body in an inappropriate way, restricting its movement. This is facilitation and the part of the spinal cord involved in it is called a facilitated segment. This is the way in which most types of lesions brought about by trauma establish themselves.

This is true in the case of a strong traumatic input into the system, although the mechanism of facilitation can occur in other ways. It always implies a constant background irritability in the nerves involved. This means that the threshold to create a nerve response is very low and needs a minimum input to trigger it. It can affect any part of the nervous system.

So facilitation can happen as a result of repetitive strain patterns of movement, chronic visceral disturbances (see the Glossary), a slight accident followed by another affecting the same area, etc. Because facilitation may provoke the inter-segmental spread of reflexes it can cause symptoms far from the site of the original problem.

CAUSES OF OSTEOPATHIC LESIONS

There are different theories about which processes in the body cause an osteopathic lesion. The majority of osteopaths, however, now believe that abnormal neurological impulses to the muscles are the most important elements. So trauma is thought to trigger abnormal nerve impulses. Trauma can be either physical as in an accident, or emotional shock — the two are not always easy to separate. Trauma may be due to repetitive movements at work — for example, playing the violin professionally. It may also come about because of poor posture, as in the case of a typist working at a word processor for hours on end.

Some problems in the internal organs of the body can disturb the other structures, and the opposite can also happen. With some cases of irritable colon, for example, the irritation can cause a contraction in the wall of the colon through reflex action in the muscles of the back thereby inducing back pain. If the normal working of any of the internal organs is disturbed over a long period of time, it may be a sign of chronic osteopathic lesion.

THE CONSEQUENCES OF LONG-STANDING OSTEOPATHIC LESIONS

The presence of an osteopathic lesion can be the cause of a number of different symptoms and disturbances of function over a period of time. The original symptoms that accompanied the lesion when it first appeared may over time change as the lesion becomes more complicated.

As symptoms may be experienced at the site of the problem and/or far away from it, it is essential to trace them back to the original cause. A series of treatments is usually needed to look at both the cause and its effects — and to solve the problem.

An example is someone with a left-sided headache, resulting from a strain of the right ankle. The strained ligaments and leg muscles cause a chain of tight muscles up the right leg and in the right side of the lower back. Subsequently, the middle of the back becomes strained because it is being overused and the reflex activity irritates the blood flow to the liver. Liver congestion causes a congestive headache. This is worse on the left side of the head because in the past the man had his left wisdom tooth taken out, leaving reduced mobility in the bones on the left side of the face and head. The pain only emerged after the whole body was decompensated because of the strained ankle.

What osteopaths call the primary lesion is what "holds" the lesion pattern, which is a series of related lesions, keeping the body unbalanced and in suffering. It may be the most important and/or the most long-standing functional problem.

The secondary lesion is the body's inappropriate response to the primary lesion. The two may be connected by the symptoms that develop over time. Think of the body as an onion with its many layers. Each layer represents a pattern of tension, the outside layers being the most recent and the deeper ones more long standing. What begins as a bad sprain of the finger and muscles of the forearm, if unresolved may in time progress to facilitation in the related nerves in the arm. A reflex irritation of the lungs, with symptoms such as a cough, wheeziness, etc., may follow.

THE OSTEOPATHIC LESION AND DISEASE

Some form of osteopathic lesion is always there where a disease takes hold and develops in the body. Correcting the lesions may be of great benefit to the sufferer, giving his body more chance to fight the disease, and helping him to function at the best possible level.

In cases like this, treatment consists of support. Someone with cancer of the liver may have bowel problems due to irritation of the nerves to the intestine, resulting in gas, colicky pains and constipation or diarrhea. Gentle treatment may be given to ease the bowel symptoms and so help the digestion.

In other cases, though, osteopathic lesions may be the underlying, predisposing factors to the disease itself. Treatment in the early stages of the problem could perhaps have prevented the disease from happening in the first place. In this way, osteopathy can be seen to have an important role in preventive medicine. Let us bear in mind that functional disorders of the type described in this chapter are the main reason why most people go to their doctor.

4

WHAT HAPPENS WHEN YOU VISIT AN OSTEOPATH?

Before describing what a patient may expect from a visit to an osteopath, let us look closely at osteopathic diagnosis and treatment.

HOW DOES AN OSTEOPATH DIAGNOSE A PROBLEM?

The first time a new patient visits an osteopath, the practitioner will try to understand the causes of the problem that has brought the person to him in the first place. A diagnosis is not written in stone — it is renewed at each visit, as the patient responds to treatment and her body changes. In time, the different layers of osteopathic lesion patterns will reveal themselves and will be treated accordingly. So the osteopath has a flexible, ongoing approach to a patient's problem.

TREATMENT

Treatment by an osteopath consists of the practical application of the principles we looked at in Chapter Two:

- the body tends naturally toward self-healing
- structure and function are interdependent
- "the rule of the artery is supreme" (the importance of good circulation of all the body fluids)
- all the parts of the body connect with each other

For each patient, the osteopath will apply these principles using the most suitable technique. As every case is unique — while the principles are universal — every patient will be treated in a very particular and specific way.

Let's take three patients, all young children complaining of the same symptoms — wheezy chest, dry cough and difficulty in breathing.

The first child had a long, difficult birth and she took her first breath with her head delivered and her body still inside the birth canal. Compression and tension remain in her chest and lungs. The second child fell off the bed, landing on her back and hitting the back of her head. Her upper back muscles contracted and her upper neck was strained, thereby irritating the vagus nerve. The third child had diffuse tension in the body and a general irritability in the nervous system with a contracted diaphragm. Sent for further tests, she was found to be allergic to cow's milk.

In all three cases the appropriate osteopathic treatment would be given to correct the structural lesions found.

THE CONSULTATION

Depending on the practitioner, you can expect your first appointment to be up to an hour long. At the end of the initial examination, the osteopath will talk to you about his findings and his suggestions for a treatment plan. During this first visit, the osteopath will not necessarily give you any treatment as such — you both need to be clear about, and to agree on, what is to be done. Before offering treatment in any case, the osteopath will evaluate whether it is appropriate for you.

The osteopath will need to know all about the problem that has brought you to his office, including exactly where the pain is, when and how it started, what makes it feel worse and what makes it feel better. He will also want to know about all your symptoms, and will ask questions in order to get as full a picture as possible. Together with information about the specific symptoms, the osteopath will want to know about your general health — if you sleep and eat well and have plenty of energy, and if there are any particular recurring problems.

There are three perspectives on what is going on when a patient arrives looking for treatment:

1. the person's personal idea about the problem

2. the practitioner's idea about the problem

3. the story that the body tells

The third will give the most accurate picture of what is happening. The body has its own memory, and is like a map of everything that has taken place in your life. The osteopath needs to have the skill to listen and observe in order to interpret what the body is telling him.

MEDICAL HISTORY

The osteopath will take a full medical history from you, finding out whether you have had a previous accident, trauma, operation or major illness such as diabetes, heart disease or cancer. In addition, the practitioner will want to know if you are presently taking any medication or have had long courses of medication in the past, or any other medical treatments.

All this information helps the osteopath to build a mind-picture of you as the patient and what you may be experiencing. Such a picture will enable him to treat you as a whole, unique individual, going beyond the apparent limits of the immediate problem.

THE EXAMINATION

As the parts and systems of the body are all interconnected, there is what an osteopath calls a mechanical logic as to why different areas develop a problem at any given time. The osteopath will give you a thorough physical examination, so you will be asked to undress to your underclothes.

The examination consists of the osteopath looking closely at your body both while you are standing, sitting and lying down. He will ask you to do some particular active movements, which will help him to see how and where you are experiencing restrictions. He will then move your spine, and other joints, while you are passive and completely relaxed, in order to feel and diagnose precisely what and where your restrictions in movement are. He will use palpation (see the Glossary) to find out which tissues are healthy and where there are painful areas.

The spine has a series of curves in it that may become straightened or even reversed; if this happens they lose their ability to absorb shock. There may also be "s" or "c" shaped curves in the spine. There are key pivot points for movement in the spine. These pivot points are points of transition and are therefore particularly vulnerable. Your chest may be expanded or contracted, your arms may hang unevenly and your pelvis may be tilted forward or backward, or be twisted. All these observations made by the practitioner will help him to understand how far you differ from what may be thought of as "normal."

Your abdomen will also be examined, and if needed, other tests such as taking your blood pressure will be done. The osteopath may also assess the involuntary mechanism (see Chapter Six).

The practitioner will then make a diagnosis and will talk to you about whether treatment is appropriate. If you agree, then treatment will go ahead.

As you have read here, on your first visit to an osteopath you will be examined thoroughly and with great care, in order for the professional to diagnose your problem accurately. A skilled practitioner is able to examine and keep evaluating a patient's condition as he monitors the effectiveness of the treatment. He also needs to be able to judge when it is necessary to refer a patient to other medical practitioners. If there is less progress than the osteopath feels there should be, he will need to re-evaluate the case or change his approach, or perhaps refer the patient elsewhere.

THE TREATMENT

The therapist never thinks of the patient as just a low-back pain case, or a migraine sufferer. In osteopathy, the patient is a whole person. As Hippocrates wrote, "It is more important to know what sort of person has the disease than to know what sort of disease the person has." The practitioner will gather as full a record as possible — as described above — of the patient's life and general state of health. She will do this through listening, observing and palpating — a continuously developing and changing process.

The ability of the osteopath to relate to her patient allows her to gain understanding of the person's problem. Mutual trust and good communication between the two people are of primary importance — a therapeutic contract is a two-way process. The techniques used by the therapist are adapted according to the person's changing physical and emotional state. The practitioner will also ask the patient to share in the treatment program by giving feedback on how he feels things are progressing.

The osteopath will not impose her own preconceived ideas on the patient, but instead will try to see the problem from *within* the unique life story of the individual. She will help the patient to identify and change those aspects of his lifestyle which may be affecting the disorder.

It is important that the contract between the practitioner and patient is quite clear. If at any time it is not, then either the patient or practitioner should feel free to call a halt to treatment. The practitioner may suggest certain conditions for treatment, which will need to be carried out by the patient if that treatment is to continue.

The main aim of the treatment is to remove the problems within the patient's body that are preventing the natural, self-healing process from taking place.

PART TWO

———

THE ART OF
OSTEOPATHY

5

OSTEOPATHIC TECHNIQUES

Osteopathic techniques are the way in which the practitioner applies the principles of osteopathy. Manual techniques are used to correct mechanical problems in the whole body; usually, a patient will be asked to relax completely while the osteopath is carrying them out. There are some techniques, though, for which an active involvement by the patient is needed and is an important part of the process.

As described in Chapter Four, the examination on the first and subsequent visits to the osteopath will show the practitioner how far his body or body part differs from the "normal." The number of techniques available to the osteopath to use in treating the lesions that may be found in the body is almost limitless. The guide for technique is the body itself. Each treatment technique is unique; it is a particular answer to any given problem in the body, because similar lesions in different people have different origins and therefore have been caused by different kinds of forces.

There are many factors that contribute to the quality of the tissue and techniques are adapted to respond to the needs of the individual. In this sense, because the tissue requirements differ from person to person and from one treatment to the next, we may say that each technique is performed only once.

Dr. Still was not especially interested in teaching techniques to his students. He always encouraged them to develop their own, using the body tissues themselves and their thorough functional anatomical knowledge as their guide. Still himself concentrated on the principles of osteopathy, developing and elaborating on them through study and through his experience.

WHAT IS "NORMAL" TISSUE?

In looking at what "normal" is for the tissues of the body, a useful starting point is a quotation from Andrew Still:

When you know the difference between normal and abnormal you have learned the all-absorbing first question: that you must take your abnormal case to the normal, lay it down, and be satisfied to leave it.

Dr. Still's interest in the laws of nature and human anatomy was profound. He wanted his students to understand how each joint and other parts of the body work, to be clear about the anatomy of the body. He believed that students of osteopathy had to be completely familiar with normal functioning, so that they could recognize the abnormal whenever they came across it in a patient.

Andrew Still did not, though, have a model of the perfect human body in his head that he wanted to impose upon patients. The norm for which he was looking was to be found within each person. In restoring balance and health to the mechanisms of the body, the osteopath is using that body as her guide; how much it can be changed or improved depends upon its own realistic limitations.

THE APPLICATION OF OSTEOPATHY

The basis for the successful application of the art of osteopathic treatment lies in the skill of palpation, which in the hands of a skillfull practitioner will make that treatment effective, painless, precise and safe.

EFFECTIVE

Treatment is effective when the osteopath responds to the needs and changes in the body tissue itself. Her skill as a practitioner will allow her to recognize what her "feeling, thinking, seeing fingers" are telling her — until such time as the expected improvement has occurred. In this way, over-treatment — which could be a cause of further irritation — will be avoided.

PAINLESS

The osteopath knows that to get the hoped for improvement, treatment should never be rushed or rough, but instead be thorough and gentle. Each movement is carried out with great care and understanding of the patient's condition.

PRECISE

The osteopath can apply her techniques precisely because of her ability to diagnose each osteopathic lesion; she can be quite specific about the exact structures that need treatment. This precision depends upon an accurate diagnosis, because without it any medical treatment can only be vague and will therefore be ineffective.

Skillfull palpation allows the osteopath to combine diagnosis and choice of techniques in a unique and accurate way.

Because of this specific approach, the greatest effect can be achieved in each treatment with the least intrusion. Sometimes following a treatment, though, the patient can experience reactions, which the osteopath will be able to anticipate and can therefore warn the patient to expect.

SAFE

What the osteopath does is entirely safe, largely because of the in-depth medical history that the practitioner takes from the patient at their first meeting. Linked with this is the thorough examination of the person. The osteopath will be aware that there may be some conditions where certain techniques are inadvisable. In the case of a patient with osteoporosis, for example, the practitioner will never use any maneuver that may cause damage to already fragile bones.

TREATMENT AND TECHNIQUE

Treatment and technique should not be thought of as the same thing. Through treatment, the osteopath has a particular goal in mind for the patient, and technique is the means to achieve this goal. The object is not just to remove symptoms, but to correct what causes them. Throughout a course of treatment, the osteopath is aware that whatever she does to one part of the body will have a bearing on the whole.

To be effective, treatment needs a plan, and the plan needs scope. So the practitioner has to have a clear aim for the overall condition of her patient. Remembering what we have said above, the aim is to restore the best possible function to the patient, specifically treating the particular condition while improving the person's general health. The techniques are the correcting maneuver used in each treatment, in order to reach the set goal. In a sense, then, we can say that the aim is both specific and general at the same time.

Treatment consists not only of manipulation and other techniques. It is also about how the osteopath relates to the patient as a fellow human being, how she is able to empathize with that person. The ability to relate to another human being and how we do this depends upon the kind of person we are, our background, our values and our own self-awareness. The relationship between the practitioner and patient is a two-way exchange of communication, requiring the osteopath to develop a deep and meaningful understanding of the patient by going beyond any preconceived ideas or judgments.

DIRECT AND INDIRECT TECHNIQUE

We have already looked at the interdependence of structure and function in the body. All osteopathic techniques involve this relationship, but in the past some have been called structural and others functional. This division into two different forms of technique no longer truly applies. All techniques are structural, because they work on the physical structure; they are also functional because they work on the function, on the job that particular structure is supposed to do within the body.

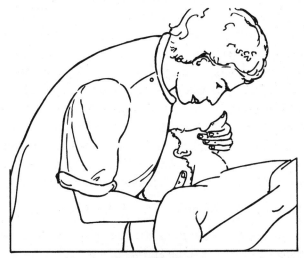

A Neck Manipulation
(rotating the third cervical vertebra to the left)

Direct technique can be applied to any part of the body in order to reverse the lesion. For example, if after a sudden turn a vertebra in the neck is twisting to the left, the osteopath will use a direct technique to turn it to the right. By contrast, indirect technique uses the body's natural responses to correct the lesion, by exaggerating whatever the restriction in movement is. A good example is how an osteopath indirectly treats an ankle joint that is twisting inward. She will very slightly encourage the ankle to twist further inward, until a point of balance is reached where the ligaments of the joint guide it back to the mid-line (where it should be).

Many of the manipulative techniques can be used either directly or indirectly. As Dr. Still said:

The osteopath must be able to use the most delicate instruments of the silversmith in adjusting the deranged, displaced bones, nerves and muscles, and remove all obstructions and thereby set the machinery of life moving.

In working with the human spine especially, the osteopath may be thought of as a musician fine-tuning an instrument. The five strings of the violin are all there, made of the finest materials; the polished wood and the pieces that connect it to those strings are fashioned with loving care. Yet without ensuring that the strings are exactly in tune, the music played will sound harsh and unpleasant to the ear. What the musician must do is to ensure that his instrument is tuned as well as possible, with a resulting harmony that is a source of great pleasure to the listener and musician alike. Likewise, the osteopath must make sure that the spine — the body's central column — and the nervous system are in tune, in order for the body to function to the best of its ability.

Following are examples of the different techniques used.

Adjustment Technique   This technique is used by many osteopaths on the spine and on other joints in the body. The diagnosis is made by examining how the joint moves, in order to see where the restrictions in movement are. The practitioner will then correct the problem by using a high velocity and low amplitude maneuver, which is usually quite painless for the patient. It is a light movement from which there may be a "cracking" sound. The movement can be used in different ways; sometimes it is used to relieve and correct a problem in just a single joint; at others it is meant to have a widespread effect.

Articulation In osteopathy, articulation involves taking the joint within its "normal" range of movement, and then gently exaggerating it if restricted.

Soft Tissue Techniques These are used on muscles and ligaments. The object is to release tightness through a form of pressure and massage.

Pumping Techniques These are mostly applied to the chest and legs and over the liver, spleen and pancreas. Their purpose is to improve circulation and drainage of waste materials. Because the organs in question are especially delicate, these techniques may need extra care on the part of the osteopath.

Muscle Energy Technique This technique involves the patient in active participation in his treatment. It can be used to correct problems in joints as well as to treat muscles. The patient is asked to contract a single muscle or group of muscles while the practitioner is gently opposing them. This opposition can be a matching force, sometimes a winning force and sometimes a losing force, depending on the case.

Traction This is a very gentle, always manual, technique. Traction is used to relieve compression or contraction in structures; it involves the osteopath pulling and stretching the appropriate area.

Osteopathic Inhibition This technique is applied to the muscles, tendons and ligaments. The osteopath uses a light pressure aimed at releasing the tissue tension. As the tissue begins to relax, the slack is taken up. The tighter the contraction, the less pressure is needed.

Functional Technique   The osteopath tests how far a joint can move — the range of its mobility — by feeling where she meets with resistance — the bind (see the Glossary). Treatment involves moving the joint in the direction which is easiest for it, until it can move freely in all directions.

Fascial Unwinding   The fascia is a slightly elastic tissue that wraps itself around all the structures in the body (see the Glossary). Unwinding the fascia involves a similar approach to functional technique as described above, except that the movement used is larger and so the response is expected from a greater spread of tissues.

Balance Ligamentous Tension   This technique is used to treat ligament strains. It follows the principles of taking the joint into its lesion pattern and then feeling the point of balance in the ligaments until a release is felt. Then the patient may be asked to inhale or exhale to exaggerate the lesion, assisting the body's self-correction. Sometimes the patient may be asked to contract a particular area and direct disengagement of the joint is used.

Working with the Primary Respiratory Mechanism (PRM) There are several techniques that can be used either directly or indirectly. Even when applied directly, the technique is always used in a very gentle way, and with a light touch on the part of the osteopath. To apply the technique indirectly means following the lesion pattern to a point of balance and stillness waiting for its release. For a more detailed explanation of the PRM, see Chapter Six.

TREATMENT OF THE VISCERA

The viscera are the important internal organs in the great cavities of the body. They include the intestines, the liver, heart, lungs, etc. Some viscera can be reached directly through gentle pressure (the abdomen, for example) as they have a muscular coat. Others cannot be reached directly, although we have developed means of treating them indirectly by contacting the surrounding structures (for example, feeling tension in and around the heart by putting your hands on the chest).

Many of the techniques outlined above can be used to treat the viscera. There is a specialized approach that has been developed in France and Belgium, which is based on the fact that there are subtle rhythms within and between organs and changes in the position of the organs. Treatment is similar to that given when working with the primary respiratory mechanism (see Chapter Six).

CONTRAINDICATIONS

The osteopath must always ensure, before starting any treatment, that there are no medical conditions that would prevent a particular patient from receiving treatment — contraindications to treatment. The medical history taken on the first visit, together with the osteopath's ability through the examination to recognize signs and symptoms for herself, should rule out any risk for the patient.

It is important to understand what is meant by "signs and symptoms." Signs are all the objective information the practitioner can obtain from taking the case history and the examination of the patient. Symptoms are the complaints from which the patient is suffering — the subjective, personal account given to the osteopath by the patient.

Suffice it to say that a skilled osteopath who is responsive to her patients, and well trained, will be aware of any potential reasons why a particular treatment should not be given to a patient.

6

THE PRIMARY RESPIRATORY MECHANISM (PRM)

The primary respiratory mechanism — first discovered by William Garner Sutherland — is a movement present throughout the body and over which we have no control. When he was a student of osteopathy in the late 1890s, while observing a disarticulated skull (that is, where the individual bones of the skull are taken apart) he was taken by the idea that the sutures or "seams" between the bones were designed to allow some movement. He noted that the articulation between the temporal and parietal bones (see the Glossary) was bevelled like the gills of a fish, and could therefore permit some kind of "breathing."

Sutherland then experimented on himself, by restricting various parts of his head. While doing this, he found within himself a range of reactions, from physiological changes throughout his body to changes in how he felt on an emotional level. Because of these reactions, Sutherland concluded that good physical and mental health depends not only on the bones of the skull being in the right position, but on the ability of the sutures to allow a slight movement. Through his research, Sutherland discovered that this movement was not confined to the head, but could be felt throughout the body, in every tissue.

Following thirty years of work on his theory, Sutherland began to teach students about this rhythmic, self-regulating movement, which he called the primary respiratory mechanism. The mechanism is characterized by the light movement of the bones of the skull and the sacrum (see the Glossary), the membrane system and the central nervous system, with the flow of the cerebrospinal fluid.

Sutherland's cranial concept, which is a detailed description of these physiological occurrences, created a new approach to osteopathic treatment and a vast range of techniques. It may in time be thought of as one of the most important discoveries in and contributions to physiology (see the Glossary).

More recent research has proven that the cranial sutures are indeed like other joints and that the head is a resilient but moving structure. At the request of the Cranial Academy (part of the American Academy of Osteopathy), the PRM has been measured by NASA physicists and numerous research papers have been published to prove its existence.

How Does the PRM Work?

The body is constantly moving and has many different rhythms, such as the heartbeat, the breathing and the waves of movement that pass food along the gut. The PRM, which is independent of all these other rhythms, is felt as an expansion and contraction of the head and body — rather as if the whole body is "breathing." There are cycles within the PRM; one cycle includes one complete expansion and contraction, and there are between eight and fourteen cycles every minute.

From time to time, the PRM stops of its own accord, and these points where there is no movement are called still points. This is when the PRM is re-balancing itself, or letting go. Osteopaths concern themselves with the rate, amplitude (that is, how fast the rhythm is and what the range of movement is) and quality of the movement, which is present at all stages of life from the newborn to the elderly. It is an indication of the level of vitality in a person, and helps the body's natural power of self-correction. Where a person has been ill or has suffered a trauma, the rate and amplitude of the PRM may be much lower than normal, or it may be absent altogether. The PRM has been seen to be the last sign of life to leave a body.

There are also other expressions of the PRM, which are characterized by their own specific rhythmicity, but it is beyond the scope of this book to go into detail.

WORKING WITH THE PRM

As a treatment approach, working with the PRM has been found to be very successful. It is also appropriate for treating patients of all ages and in all states of health.

The principles of working with the PRM are taught to osteopaths training at undergraduate level, although most of the in-depth study is done by osteopaths who have completed their basic training. To work with the PRM, the osteopath must have the capacity to be increasingly still within himself. Working with it fits perfectly with the osteopathic principle of the practitioner as an assistant to the internal, self-healing power of the body.

Today, after years of observation and building up evidence on the PRM, reasons have been found for numerous symptoms and conditions that have long puzzled practitioners in all forms of healing. Now, orthodox doctors, ophthalmologists, obstetricians, gynecologists and specialists from fields as diverse as dentistry and psychotherapy are becoming knowledgeable about the PRM, and are increasingly collaborating with osteopaths.

THE PRM AND TREATMENT

During treatment, a patient will usually feel only a very light pressure from the practitioner's hands, and many of the techniques require a very gentle touch indeed. The osteopath's hands may be placed on the head, spine or sacrum, as well as on an arm or leg or over an organ such as the liver. With complicated cases, two osteopaths may work

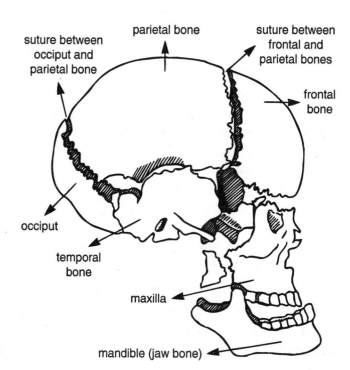

A Disarticulated Skull

parietal bone

suture between occiput and parietal bone

suture between frontal and parietal bones

frontal bone

occiput

temporal bone

maxilla

mandible (jaw bone)

together on the same patient, one for example taking the head and the other the pelvis.

Exaggeration or Indirect Technique

In this form of treatment, the practitioner's hands gently exaggerate the tensions felt in whatever tissue is being worked on, so that the hands actually become a support for the distortion itself. When a point of balance is reached, the patient's own self-healing, self-correcting power will use it as a "mirror" to guide the structure back to an appropriate "neutral" position.

This approach is the most commonly used one, although not on small children or adult patients in cases where there is great trauma. In those instances, a direct technique will be used. There are also other treatment methods that are not explained here.

The Effects of Treatment

Most treatments take place while the patient is lying down, although some techniques are more effective when the person is sitting up.

Treatment is often a deeply relaxing experience, which allows the patient to quieten the conscious mind to a point where she can concentrate her attention on her own inner resources. The patient may experience a change in her breathing as the restrictions in the body are released. People are often aware of what is happening in one part of their body, while the osteopath's hands are placed some distance away; this is due to the fact that, as outlined earlier in the book, everything in the body is connected.

The functional unity of the body is created by the neuro-endocrine-immune system, closely linked to the circulatory system. In a different way, the fascia forms a continuous connection throughout the whole body, as do muscle chains (see the Glossary). So by working specifically on one of these systems, the others may be influenced.

Patients often sense that their body has been truly heard, and healed. Others may not be aware of anything in particular happening during treatment, although they appreciate that they do feel different afterward and are getting better. The changed sensations that a patient may feel during and immediately after treatment may last for hours, a day or a week, but the deeper physiological effects will continue for a considerable time.

WHO AND WHAT PROBLEMS CAN BE HELPED?

Osteopathic treatment using the primary respiratory mechanism can also be given when other treatment techniques may not be suitable for a patient. Because this approach is particularly gentle, it is therefore appropriate for the following groups of people:

- newborn babies
- young children
- pregnant women
- women who have passed menopause
- people who are in a lot of pain or who cannot be moved
- immediately after surgery
- people with complicated medical histories
- the elderly
- the terminally ill

Osteopathic treatment using the PRM is not a "cure all." For people with long-term or complicated illness, the osteopath will recommend that the patient should have additional help — from a medical herbalist, an Alexander teacher (see the Glossary) or some other specialist such as a surgeon, for example.

Some of the most common conditions that can be helped are:

- bowel or bladder problems where the organ is not functionally properly
- ear inflammations that are not infectious
- congested or red eyes
- dental problems such as malalignment of the jaws
- jaw pain
- migraine
- neuralgia
- sinusitis
- strains of the muscles and ligaments

This is by no means an exhaustive list, and many other complaints can also be helped in this way.

What Can Damage the PRM?

Trauma such as may happen in a difficult birth, a whiplash injury, blows to the head, falls on to the base of the spine and dental extractions can interfere with the movement inherent in the primary respiratory mechanism. This movement may also be influenced by shock after a major accident or operation, after a serious infection, fever or emotional shock. Poor nutrition, food additives, drugs, toxins, heavy metals and pollutants in our water and air — such as lead from exhaust fumes — also slow the PRM down. When this happens, the bones of the head and sacrum tend to lock, giving a hard feel to the osteopath's hands as he examines the patient.

A trauma can compress the tissues, stopping the motion that normally takes place in that part of the body. This results in stagnation and means that even the micromotion of these cells is affected; the usual, constant flow of fluid is interrupted and so the workings of the body are altered.

Bearing in mind that all the cells in the body have a "memory" (see Chapter Two) the echo of trauma may remain locked in a part of the body for many years, acting as an anchor on the person's vitality and energy. In cases where there is extreme trauma, the PRM can actually stop completely, and so the individual becomes progressively more seriously ill, on a downward spiral.

In those who are clinically depressed or mentally ill, the movement is slower than in other people.

WHAT IS HEALING?

The body makes so many demands upon itself that sometimes full healing does not take place. Where an acute problem has been "cured," we often forge ahead with our lives, but with a low level of injury still present. During osteopathic treatment, problems at this level can be brought back to the body's attention, so that they can be fully healed. After a leg has been fractured and the bone has been repaired, for example, it may still ache in damp weather and feel like it is not a fully functioning part of the rest of the body. The osteopath will check whether the PRM is in the bone, as it should be; if it is not, with the right technique the practitioner will be able to restore it so that the bone can "breathe" again.

As mentioned above, treatment may or may not give fast relief. More recent injuries will respond more easily than long-standing ones, and the younger the patient the speedier the response. With long-term problems, it may take several months of regular treatment to achieve a lasting change.

People who have been in discomfort for a long time may find it difficult to be patient. The osteopath will have to ask them to bear with it and wait for results; these will depend on the patient's level of energy, general state of health, specific condition and the practitioner's understanding of their individual problem.

EMOTIONAL HEALING

Osteopathic treatment has been found to benefit people emotionally as well as physically. Stress, fear and anxiety can interfere with the breathing and therefore reduce the oxygen intake to the lungs. If the distress is considerable, or lasts for some time, it may also interfere with the normal movement of the primary respiratory mechanism, which in itself will increase the person's anxiety.

Tension in the chest may be caused by heart-felt feelings of loss or grief. The release of what an osteopath calls these "holding patterns" of tension may also allow such emotions to come to the surface and be consciously expressed. This can create a new sense of joy and well-being and other positive feelings that have been blocked perhaps for some time.

During treatment, there are times when the patient may benefit from talking frankly and openly about her life.

HEALING THE WHOLE PERSON

The changes that happen in serious conditions are complicated. In addition, because the healing process involves the whole person, it is the "whole" that needs to be treated and understood. For this reason, the collaboration between healthcare professionals that we referred to earlier in the book is essential. It is equally important not to look for a single "magic pill" to cure all problems, although some modern medicines of course have a very useful specific application that can be invaluable.

Because there are always unknown factors within each individual, which seem to take the person beyond their own limitations, there are cases in which some people have been healed from conditions that had been diagnosed as terminal (such as cancer). Cases like these represent moments of deep healing, marked by a total transformation in the person. The changes involve not only their physical, mental and emotional being, but also the web of their relationships with family, work and the world around them.

We believe that health is crucially linked to a flexibility and ability to change, the responsibility for which lies largely within each of us.

PART THREE

—

HEALING WITH OSTEOPATHY

7

PREGNANCY, CHILDBIRTH, AND CHILDREN

Today, osteopathy is best known as a treatment for back pain, and many people think of it as a system of medicine that specializes in problems associated with the muscles and the bones. Increasingly, though, the public is realizing that osteopathy can benefit many other conditions, and that it can be a very suitable treatment for pregnant women, young babies and children. The case studies in Chapter Nine clearly show the range of conditions, for people of all ages, that can be helped by receiving treatment from an osteopath.

PREGNANCY

At no other time in a woman's life does her body undergo so many changes as during pregnancy. The ligaments soften and yield, the curves of the spine change and the posture is altered. Because of the weight of the baby, the center of gravity in the expectant mother gradually moves forward, which often creates an arching in the lower back and therefore an increase in the spinal curves. This is most noticeable in the last three months of pregnancy.

The strain in the spine at this time is likely to be greatest on the lumbar and dorsal vertebrae (see the Glossary). Symptoms such as nausea and heartburn can arise because of tension in the diaphragm and solar plexus and because of the restrictions on the related areas of the spine. Circulatory problems, such as swelling of the legs and varicose veins, may be the result of increased pressure in the abdomen. General swelling may be caused by pressure on the kidneys, and similarly sciatica and changes in bladder and bowel habits may result. All of these problems can be helped by osteopathic treatment.

Treatment given during pregnancy is very gentle and quite safe. It is a good time to have it, in fact, as the body is changing so much and so quickly. Any existing restrictions or strains can be released relatively easily because the ligaments are softer than usual.

PREVENTION

It is advisable for any woman who has suffered from a bad back and is considering becoming pregnant to visit an osteopath for a thorough check-up. Any existing restrictions in the spine can then be treated, and the whole body helped to find its optimum balance. Such preventive measures should result in a more comfortable pregnancy and an easier delivery (see below).

CHILDBIRTH

For a woman to have the easiest labor possible, her pelvic and lower back joints need to be free-moving. The automatic process of birth — basically a series of reflexes — can be hampered if there are any restrictions in the relevant joints. Similarly there can be difficulties if the woman has had problems with how the visceral organs (see the Glossary) function, or if the muscle tone in the pelvic region is not as it should be. Any past problems, such as falls, operations, infections and emotional shocks can remain locked in the memory of the tissues for years to come. In safe, skilled hands, any such lingering difficulties can be recognized and treated.

During the birth, the baby's head and body are put under great stress and compression, which can stay within the tissues throughout childhood and into later life. As the baby is pushed through the birth canal, the head and upper neck are especially under pressure. At this stage, the bones are fairly soft and some are still in parts, not having yet formed one single bone.

Moulding, where the bones of the skull overlap to ease the baby's passage into the world, happens during the birth. Moulding can also happen because the baby drops down into a low position in the womb in the last weeks before the birth. It is usually corrected afterward by the baby's crying and the pressure of the tongue on the roof of the mouth during breast-feeding. Sometimes, if the forces on the head are very strong or prolonged, the moulding remains and can cause problems.

Another area that takes much of the strain during the birth is where the upper cervical spine (see the Glossary) joins the skull. This area is very important in terms of the nervous system; the baby's ability to hold his head up and to suck depends on the freedom of movement here. If the baby is born prematurely, these parts of the body are even more vulnerable.

According to research by Dr. Viola Fryman, in a study of 1,500 newborn babies, nine out of ten suffered trauma while being born. Babies can safely receive treatment from an osteopath within hours of the birth. While the tissues are still soft, it is a good idea for both mother and baby to have an examination soon after the delivery.

DIFFICULT BIRTHS

A difficult labor can happen because of a number of different things. It may be too long, or too fast, when the baby is expelled out of the birth canal very quickly. Trauma can result from the use of forceps or ventouse extraction (see the Glossary). Trauma can also come from a breech delivery, or where the baby's face is facing forward, or where the mother has a cesarean section. The umbilical cord is sometimes wrapped around the baby's neck, in which case there can be tension in the baby's neck and abdomen; this can also happen if the cord is cut before it stops pulsating. A memory of trauma may remain in the tissues if the baby takes his or her first breath when the head is out but the shoulders were stuck, so that the lungs were not able to expand fully.

HOW TO SPOT PROBLEMS IN THE NEWBORN

Symptoms to be aware of in the newborn baby are:

- colic
- constipation or diarrhea
- continuous crying
- difficulty in feeding, or preferring to feed from one side
- excessive gas
- gummy eyes
- nervousness
- restless sleep (or too much sleep)
- stiffness in the muscles of the neck (torticollis)

It is hard for a new parent to know what would be too much or too little sleep, as each baby is so different. A guideline, though, may be between sixteen to twenty hours sleep a day, with wakeful periods in the day and night. If the sleeping pattern is excessively beyond these limits, and especially if there are other symptoms present as mentioned above, it is a good idea to have your baby checked by an osteopath.

Likewise, babies have little control over their necks and neck muscles for some time, making it difficult for a new parent to know if there are problems. Perhaps the simplest, and best, question to ask yourself is: "Does my baby seem comfortable?"

All the symptoms above may be caused by strain in the body, left over from the birth, particularly in the baby's head. In functional torticollis, for example, which is caused by a contracted muscle in the neck, the nerve that serves the muscle may be trapped due to compression in the bones that make up the skull. By gently working to free it, the osteopath can allow the problem to resolve itself.

As mentioned above, one of the most valuable ways in which an osteopath can help the newborn baby is by restoring the structure of the head and body to balanced alignment right after the birth. This is preventive osteopathic medicine at its best. See "Case Studies," Case Two.

CHILDREN

Dr. Sutherland, a student of Dr. Still, used a very apt expression to describe how strain in children's heads can grow into strain in adults' heads: "As the twig is bent so doth the tree incline." There are many grown-ups who would not be suffering from the same problems if they had had appropriate treatment as children.

Children go to an osteopath with a range of symptoms and conditions, including the following:

- asthma

- coordination difficulties

- dental problems

- digestive problems

- dyslexia

- glue ear

- hyperactivity

- speech problems

- scoliosis (abnormal curving of the spine)

Children are very delicate in comparison with adults, and so osteopathic treatment has to be adapted to suit the needs of the young body. Correcting strains at a young age allows

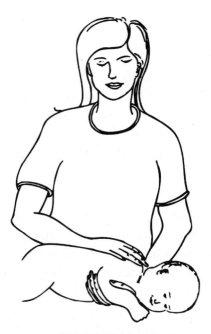

Baby Being Treated
(assisting the primary respiratory mechanism)

the child to reach and express his full potential as a unique person.

Scoliosis, mentioned above in the list of symptoms and conditions, is a complicated problem where osteopathic care is of great importance. This applies not only to trying to prevent the condition from happening in the first place, but also for managing it if it has become established. The majority of scoliosis cases begin as functional disturbances of the musculoskeletal system.

BRAIN-DAMAGED CHILDREN

There are many problems that children suffer from, such as cerebral palsy, autism and epilepsy, that can benefit from osteopathic treatment.

Cerebral palsy covers a wide range of symptoms. The damage done to the body is not usually progressive, although the symptoms may change over time. Minor symptoms include slight spasticity in an arm or leg, uncoordinated movement and learning difficulties. More severe symptoms can be a lack of control over the posture, an inability to move without help, seizures, eye and ear problems and mental retardation. The cause of such damage is by no means clear, though it is accepted that a difficult birth has a considerable bearing on the child's growth and development.

CENTRAL NERVOUS SYSTEM

Osteopaths believe that where there is brain damage in a child, there is also an error in the inherent involuntary movement in the central nervous system. The brain matures rapidly in the first year of life, and a great deal can be done in this respect if treatment begins very soon after birth.

Osteopathy cannot restore function to dead neurons (see the Glossary). However, treatment to restore the movement that should be present in the central nervous system helps to free the brain to do the best job it can in whatever the circumstances. It is not easy to give an answer when parents ask how far their child can be helped. An osteopath cannot give false hope, but it is important for the practitioner and the parents to keep an open but realistic mind about the outcome. Every child responds differently, depending on his or her personal story, but with osteopathic treatment almost all cases show some improvement in the quality of life.

8

OSTEOPATHY
AND DENTISTRY

———

Dentists and osteopaths are working together more and more nowadays. This makes a great deal of sense, because there is a fundamental relationship between proper, balanced movement in the face and mouth and in the rest of the body. In other words, there is a body attached to the head! The connection between the position of the teeth when the jaw is closed (occlusion) and how osteopathy can influence this by working on the head and body as a whole is very complicated.

Sometimes a common toothache may be due to a problem of restricted movement in the upper part of the neck. An overstimulated nerve in this area irritates the nerves in the face.

Most people think that the skull and face are made up of bones that do not move. From the observation and work of skilled osteopaths, however, it is clear that the head is instead a dynamic and mobile structure. All the bones in the cranium are designed to move, or "breathe," slightly — the primary respiratory mechanism or PRM (see Chapter Six). The sutures joining the bones together are like moveable hinges, allowing a gentle spreading; this gives a pumping action to the system, without which it will not work as it should.

DISTORTION OF THE JAWS (MALOCCLUSION)

Your dentist is concerned with the size, shape and relationship of your teeth so that they fit together properly. Underdevelopment or distortion of one or both jaws and therefore the teeth are well recognized in dentistry. Corrections are made by directly straightening teeth and widening the arch between the jaws by using various kinds of braces.

We need our jaws to fit together well to have healthy gums and teeth. The joints and soft tissues that work the jaw also depend on this. If all is as it should be, we can talk, chew and grind without causing any problems.

The ligament that attaches the tooth to its socket is called the peridontal ligament. It is highly sensitive and richly supplied with nerve fibers. This is how we are aware of even the smallest variation of pressure on each tooth — remember what it feels like to have a piece of celery string caught between your teeth! This sensitivity shows how important it is to have even contact between the teeth.

SIGNS OF MALOCCLUSION

There are a number of clear signs and symptoms that show problems in how a person's jaws fit together. Among these are heavily worn down teeth, shiny spots or grooves on fillings and teeth that are not straight in the jaw. The patient may also have had problems with broken teeth or fillings; clenching or grinding the teeth (especially at night); white lines in the mouth; and scalloped edges to the tongue.

Malocclusion can begin with a difficult birth, as we looked at in the previous chapter. Inherited problems such as too many or too few teeth, a blow to the face or jaw or poor diet can also create difficulties. Even where it looks like a child may have inherited some problems, though, there are likely to be other factors that could benefit from osteopathic treatment. Ideally, treatment should begin as soon as possible after the birth.

BIRTH TRAUMA AND MALOCCLUSION

It has been known for some time that many problems that dentists are called upon to deal with are developmental, and may in part be caused by difficulties during the birth of a baby. Osteopathic work with the primary respiratory mechanism has further recognized the significance of such trauma. The process of being born can sometimes compress the head, and such babies may have asymmetric faces and unusually high palates.

Some of the following symptoms in an infant or young child can suggest such problems:

- allergies
- behavioral or learning difficulties
- recurrent ear infections
- eye problems
- hyperactivity
- nasal symptoms
- difficulties in swallowing

Habits such as breathing through the mouth, thumb-sucking, biting the lips, sleeping only on one side of the face and early or late loss of milk teeth are all effects, not causes.

If the compressions are treated early enough, the results may be two-fold: immediate release of the restriction; and a gradual re-moulding of the abnormalities in the structure of the jaws. The best insurance against future malcurvature of the spine and malocclusion is when the osteopath removes the restrictions in the newborn that prevent the normal movement of the PRM in the head.

Other Causes of Malocclusion

Direct trauma to the jaw and face can also cause problems. Falling forward on to chin and blows to the jaw can distort the temporomandibular joints (see the Glossary) and compress the bones of the face and head. Having teeth out can also leave unwelcome forces between and inside the bones of the mouth and face, so if possible avoid having any teeth removed — unless it is absolutely necessary.

If some teeth are missing, or only one side of the mouth is used for chewing, an unequal and considerable strain is placed on one joint.

The cheek bones continue to grow throughout your life. So where a person's teeth are all removed and dentures fitted, there may be bone loss in the face over a period of time. The dentures may therefore need to be built up to compensate for this. If the dentures are the wrong height, they may create an imbalance in the jaw muscles.

The Importance of Treatment

There are direct connections between the alignment of the teeth, the symmetry of the joints, the curves in the spine, the levels of the shoulder blades and pelvis, and leg length. You can see this for yourself if you wear an inappropriate heel lift in your shoe for just a day; afterward there may be discomfort in the areas that are connected.

It is important for those who have malocclusion to have their whole bodies examined by an osteopath. If the problems in the jaw are solved, then many other connected problems can also be helped. Among these are:

- backache

- breathing difficulties

- deteriorating eyesight

- headaches

- hormonal problems

- painful teeth

- sinusitis

- scoliosis

Effect of Orthodontic Treatment

An orthodontist is a dentist who specializes in correcting malocclusion. It often happens, even after years of the best orthodontic treatment available, that when the brace is removed the problems in a patient's jaw return. This is obviously very disappointing to the patient, the parents and the orthodontist, who has given the most appropriate treatment in his experience.

The basic problem lies in the fact that when a brace is fitted in a mouth where there are misalignments, the brace itself simply adds to the compression already present. The brace may even introduce new restrictions that were not there before. With the change in alignment brought about by the brace, altered pressures will be put on the teeth, the sinuses and the soft tissues, which may restrict growth. So it is important while such dental work is being done that the patient is regularly checked out by the osteopath, even where there are no apparent problems. These regular check-ups should continue after the orthodontic treatment has finished until the situation is stable.

If there is free movement within the jaw and face before the orthodontist begins his course of corrective treatment, he will only have to encourage the bones and the teeth into the positions that they are ready to accept. The PRM itself will adapt to the changes and the corrected position of the jaw will be secure when the treatment is over. The orthodontic treatment itself will then be easier and less uncomfortable.

Sometimes dramatic changes in the way the upper and lower jaws fit together can be achieved merely by restoring normal, free motion within the head and face.

9

CASE STUDIES

The following case studies will show you how the theory and principles of osteopathic treatment are applied in practice. The range of patients treated also illustrates how suitable osteopathy can be for treating young and older people alike.

CASE ONE

Lucy is a thirty-nine-year-old mother, who came in for osteopathic treatment when she was two months pregnant with her second child. She complained of tiredness; discomfort at the base of her neck; headaches on the right side; and pain in the lower back when she awoke in the morning.

Lucy had suffered two serious accidents in the past. The first was at thirteen years old, when she fell and broke her chin on the right side. The second was a fall from her horse at the age of sixteen, when she landed on her sacrum, resulting in a crush fracture of the second lumbar vertebra.

Her first pregnancy and birth had gone very well, without complications, although during the delivery of the baby Lucy had felt some sciatic pain in the right leg.

TREATMENT

Treatment was given to release the tension in Lucy's right shoulder muscles, which were clearly tighter than those on the left. Her spine between the shoulder blades and in the mid-lower back was restored to normal movement where it had been rigid. The compression retained in the bone of the fractured vertebra and mandible (see the Glossary) was released to allow full expression of the PRM.

Lucy received treatment twelve times in all, regularly throughout her pregnancy. A number of techniques were used in Lucy's case, such as: inhibition to the contracted muscles; balanced ligamentous tension release of the right clavicle joints; manipulation to the mid-back; and a variety of gentle techniques to encourage movement in the cranium and sacrum.

OUTCOME

After the first few treatments, the pain in her lower back eased, she felt less tired and the headaches disappeared.

Two weeks before the baby was born the old symptom of sciatic pain in the right leg came back, but it eased again after a couple of treatments. Pain around Lucy's right ear, which had been a feature of her headaches, also returned. This pain also cleared after two treatments.

Lucy was given advice on what to do just before or during delivery should the pain return. We suggested massaging her right buttock and gently stretching her lower back muscles (both standing and lying down) just before delivery.

On the day of the birth Lucy's husband was stranded by poor weather in another town some distance away. Lucy felt considerable anxiety about this, and although the birth was easy it was more painful than her first, with sciatica. However, she recovered quickly, with no other symptoms, and the baby is doing well.

CASE TWO

Louis was five weeks old when he was brought to us with colic, gas and an inflamed rash around his genitals. He was not sleeping soundly between feedings, and instead was restless, groaning and holding his lifted knees up to his chest while contracting his tummy muscles.

Louis was his mother Sarah's first child. Sarah had had problems in the last stage of labor, with the baby's head emerging and then receding several times; he also had the umbilical cord wrapped around his neck. Finally Louis was born with help from the doctor, who pressed down on Sarah's stomach. She tore in the process, needing four stitches.

Immediately after the birth Louis' head appeared flattened and squashed at the front and he did not want to be touched. He slept for nine hours, after which he began to feed.

Sarah recalled that during the last few weeks of pregnancy she had felt the baby's head descend low into her pelvis, pushing on her pubic bone.

THE EXAMINATION

Louis' eyes appeared to be squashed by the low position of his forehead and his right eye was sticky. His primary respiratory mechanism was less fluid in movement than it should have been and the sacrum was jammed between the ilia (see the Glossary).

TREATMENT

Louis received five treatments in total. These consisted of easing the jammed sacrum, unwinding the tension in his tummy, releasing a compression in the center of his chest and freeing his upper neck by using balanced ligamentous tension.

Outcome

After the third treatment, Louis' pelvis "shuddered" and he sighed as his sacrum was released from the position it had been trapped in. Over the next few days his rash cleared and he began sleeping for longer periods of time. The later treatments were aimed at lifting his frontal bone, after which his right eye became clear.

Clearly Louis was a strong baby and basically quite well. However, his body had retained some of the classic signs of strain from the last weeks of his mother's pregnancy and his birth into the world.

Case Three

Nine-year-old Sam was brought to us by his mother because of his difficulty in concentrating and a squint. Both Sam's eyes tended to turn inward, particularly the left one. He was wearing glasses to help correct the problem.

When he was one year old, Sam suffered from pneumonia and six months later he hit his right temple when he fell from his mother's bicycle. At the age of six he fractured his left forearm and at nine years of age he fractured the right one.

The muscles of Sam's left eye were operated on when he was seven, though a few months later the eye was turning inward as before. Sam was self-conscious and very anxious to get rid of his squint.

Sam fidgeted constantly, not concentrating when answering questions and bumped into furniture all the time.

THE EXAMINATION

When we examined Sam, we found restrictions in his spine, at the base of his neck and between his shoulder blades. His head had a series of strains and there was compression both around the eyes and around the back of his head (the occiput).

TREATMENT

Sam had five treatments initially, and continued to have monthly treatments for three months following improvements in his condition.

The techniques used were aimed at increasing the PRM (see Chapter Six) in Sam's neck. One light manipulation was used to the vertebra at the base of the neck, which was very jammed. A sideway shift of the forehead was gently eased into alignment. The underside of this bone forms part of the

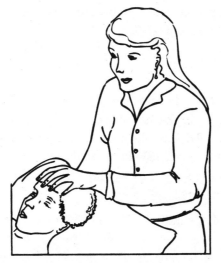

A Cranial Hold
(contacting the front and back of the head to release
the membranes inside the head)

bony eye socket where the muscles that control eye movement attach. So this realignment also released tension within the eye socket.

OUTCOME

During the third treatment, Sam became completely still for the first time. This happened at the same time as an increased voluntary movement in his head. After this treatment, Sam's mother noticed that he became more able to concentrate and his school teachers commented on how changed he was.

Continuing treatment further released his eye muscles, improving Sam's squint. His mother said that most of the time his eye was straight, turning inward only when he was tired or upset. He had a check-up with the optician two months after osteopathic treatment began to discuss the possibility of another operation. The optician was very pleased, deciding not to operate but to wait for another year (with the intention that if a second operation is performed it may have a more lasting effect).

CASE FOUR

Sarah, aged fourteen, came for treatment complaining of headaches, backache (in the lower back), pain in her legs and very flat feet. Her mother was concerned because the orthopedic specialist she had consulted wanted to operate on Sarah's feet to increase the arch, in order to improve her whole posture.

During her childhood Sarah had a number of problems. At four years of age she had her appendix removed and at five she had her adenoids taken out. At the age of seven and a half she began to get severe headaches on the right side of her head. At ten, Sarah had spent one month in the hospital with peritonitis.

A removable brace had been on Sarah's teeth for a year to widen her palate and to straighten three teeth that were distorted (this had not made the headaches worse). Her dentist intended to move the teeth around in the lower jaw so that the upper and lower jaws and teeth would meet as they should.

THE EXAMINATION

During the examination restrictions were found in the joints of the upper neck and the dorsal spine (see the Glossary) between the shoulder blades. Sarah's posture was poor, with her shoulders drooping forward and a long sway back (that is, her back had a long, shallow lumbar curve).

While standing, Sarah had a lot of tension in her leg muscles and a contraction in the right side of her abdomen. The muscles and joints on the left side of her head and face were restricted. The whole lower jaw was shifted to the left and the muscles that attach the jaw to the head were very tight and tender on that side.

TREATMENT

Treatment was aimed at mobilizing the restricted joints in her spine and upper neck and inhibiting the contracted muscle in the abdomen. The jaw was "unwound" (see Chapter Five) on several occasions. Specific work was also done to release the compressed joints on the side of Sarah's face, using the PRM found in the examination. Sarah was also given an exercise to relax her jaw.

Sarah received seven treatments at increasing intervals of time. She was then advised to return after the brace had been removed.

OUTCOME

With increased mobility in her head and face Sarah's headaches disappeared. Her lower back and legs also became more comfortable and so her mother decided not to go ahead with the operation.

CASE FIVE

Fred, a thirty-five-year-old goldsmith, came with low back pain that started when he was aged thirty, following an operation on his right knee. The pain took the form of a general ache across his lower back, involving the right sacro-iliac joint. Since the operation Fred had had no further problems with his knee. Six months before visiting us, he had had a stiff neck for several days, and difficulty in turning his head to the left.

Over the years, Fred suffered from a number of medical problems. At the age of twelve he suffered from inflammation of the tendon below the right kneecap. At twenty-five he had an operation to remove a stone from his right kidney. From then on he noticed that if he did not drink a minimum amount of water each day his urine became opaque. He fell on his neck while skiing when he was thirty. X-rays were taken of Fred's whole spine before his knee operation. These showed slight scoliosis, a loss of cervical curve and reduced disc space between the fifth lumbar vertebra and the sacrum.

Fred had received chiropractic treatment every six months for several years. The practitioner had worked mostly on Fred's sacrum and pelvic joints, which were very rigid. Fred had also taken lessons in the Alexander technique (see the Glossary).

FAMILY BACKGROUND

Fred's mother suffered from low back pain since she was thirty years of age; one sister was diagnosed as having scoliosis at thirteen, and the other two sisters also had low back pain.

THE EXAMINATION

The osteopathic examination revealed that Fred's whole spine was generally "stiff," with a lack of movement in the vertebral joints at the level of the upper dorsal spine (see the Glossary). His right shoulder was held higher than the left, and the head bent slightly to the left side. There were a series of restrictions in the lower part of his body. The right hip was held in relatively more internal rotation, the right psoas (see the Glossary) was contracted and the right kidney was held inferiorly.

We recommended that Fred have a scan of his right kidney and urine analysis; he did this, and both showed no problems.

TREATMENT

Fred had treatment over four months. The treatment was at first aimed at releasing the tension in his spine, by working directly on the tight joints and contracted muscles. After five sessions, Fred felt some immediate relief in his lower back that never lasted more than three days. When the lower back felt better a new pain appeared in his upper back and neck.

Fred felt quite depressed about it, and told us that he feared his problem was caused by a combination of hereditary factors and the knee operation. He doubted it could change.

During the next session we decided to work together as a team. While we were working on a compression of the fascia in Fred's chest he had an emotional release where he cried for the first time in many years about a problem in a close relationship. After this treatment Fred's whole spine "softened" and became less stiff. The pain in his lower and upper back disappeared, but an older pain that he had experienced before his right knee operation came back. The knee swelled and locked. Fred found it quite difficult to walk because of the resulting stiffness in the right leg.

Fred arrived at the next treatment session quite angry, worried about taking time off work and confused about re-experiencing the old problem. Local treatment was given to his right knee, hip and psoas muscle and he was advised to use hot and cold packs on the knee. In a week the knee had cleared and Fred continued to improve. We explained the importance of going on to treat his lower back and kidney to ensure that it was able to move freely. Fred agreed to continue treatment for a while longer.

LEARNING FROM THE CASE

Fred was open to our osteopathic explanations about his reactions to treatments and put his trust in us. This is very important for a successful outcome.

The reactions Fred experienced during treatment may be explained by the idea that the body stores its experiences in layers, with the most recent problem in the "uppermost" layer and problems from further back in the past in the "underneath" layers. When he first came to us the most evident tension was in his upper back, even though Fred was aware of discomfort in his lower back. When this area was released it revealed the underlying problem, which was unresolved strain left over from the knee operation and possibly some referred pain irritation from the right kidney. Sometimes we can compensate for a part of the body that is not working properly by shifting the problem elsewhere.

If a problem is held in the body for long enough it can go into deeper levels. It has long been observed that in many cases of visceral disease the pain is not felt in the organ itself but is referred to the musculoskeletal system, often far from the site of the original problem. Some kinds of kidney disease produce intense pain in the lower back and groin. Through the same nerve pathways prolonged contracture of muscles and ligaments may cause a reflex irritation to the viscera.

In Fred's case, the first trauma was apparently an inflamed right knee at twelve years of age followed by an operation for a kidney stone at the age of twenty-five. The fact that the chiropractor had worked a great deal on Fred's pelvis suggested also, however, that there was perhaps previous deep contracture and restriction in that area. It is difficult to say which came first at this moment in time, but we can see links between the knee, the pelvis and the kidney. The body may deposit calcium in tissues that do not move freely. We do not know what disturbed Fred's kidney, but clearly at the age of twenty-five it was not working well and had obvious restrictions.

OUTCOME

After the course of treatment, Fred's back and neck felt better than they had in years. Several months later, after spending a day on the beach and in the evening getting a chill, the low back pain and stiffness returned in a less intense form. On examination, the right lower back muscles were tender and contracted. After two treatments Fred felt better, with only some stiffness when standing still.

Fred has become aware that part of the problem is a feeling of fear of his back getting blocked, which seems to contribute to the tension.

CASE SIX

Lisa was brought to us by her mother when she was two-and-a-half years old. Lisa's birth was induced because she was a week overdue and her mother's amniotic fluid was dark when it broke. According to the Apgar score (see the Glossary), Lisa was quite normal in every respect. At birth she was also lively and pink, but she had inhaled some meconium (see the Glossary) and had a slight rattle in her chest. Her mother Sandra's pregnancy had been good, except that in the fifth month Sandra had contractions; a stitch was sewn in her cervix to keep the baby in place.

Lisa was given oxygen and had a routine procedure to help her breathe, during which she began to have an irregular heartbeat. After eight hours, Lisa was transferred to another hospital and was treated with medication and put into an incubator. Over subsequent days, chest X-rays and an electrocardiogram showed that the left side of her heart was enlarged.

Lisa spent the first three months of her life in intensive care and left the hospital when she was eight months old. During this time Lisa had a number of medical problems, including digestive difficulties, vomiting and an inflammation of the upper right lobe of her lung. Lisa also had several operations, including a tracheotomy and a blood transfusion.

A brain scan at seven months showed that Lisa's development was considerably behind what was expected for that age and she also had drooping eyelids. At the age of two she had surgery — partially successful — to correct her eyelids. Overall, Lisa's prognosis was poor.

Lisa was still small for her age at two-and-a-half and not really able to open her eyes properly. She was able to crawl and sit up, but preferred to be lying down. She was not talking at all, and seemed very much dependent on her mother. Closed in her own little world, Lisa was very shy of men, including her father. Her parents have two other healthy children, both older than Lisa.

Lisa had been treated twice a week by a physiotherapist and was seeing a neuropsychologist three times a year. She had seen an osteopath occasionally for a year after she came out of the hospital, and from that time her head started to grow more. She had recently started to attend a playgroup three mornings a week.

Her mother was particularly worried about the fact that Lisa's head still seemed small for her age. She was concerned about her ongoing constipation, colds with excessive mucous from the sinuses and upper respiratory tract and her reduced vision. Lisa was very sensitive to sound, although she often actively sought out noises.

THE EXAMINATION

From observation, Lisa's development was comparable to that of an eight-month-old baby. She arched her head and spine backward, had a series of involuntary movements with her head and hands, uttered only guttural sounds and was very attracted to bright light.

On examination, our findings included a compression of the central nervous system and of the skull and tension in the membranes, especially around the head. Lisa's spine was held rigidly from the end of the upper dorsal vertebra down to the sacrum. The colon and the throat were contracted, with the tracheotomy hole still there. The joints of Lisa's arms and legs were much more mobile than normal.

TREATMENT

Lisa was seen every two weeks for six months, then once a month, and treatment continues on a monthly basis. Our aim is to release the shock and compression within the central nervous system and the head.

OUTCOME

Lisa is now three-and-a-half years old. She walks, plays and makes a range of sounds. She also goes willingly into her father's arms and wants to be involved in the life going on around her. She seems to enjoy music and is very curious, but unless encouraged by an adult, Lisa will not play in a small group of children except when they sing a song she enjoys or play "ring around the roses." Lisa mostly plays alone.

She still appears to be easily frightened and very sensitive, although more able to communicate what she wants. She already shows signs of being aware of the difference between herself and other children, being rather defensive at times.

Lisa's last brain scan showed significant changes — large parts of the brain that were previously immature were now seen to have developed normally. The brain as a whole still looked rather small for a child of Lisa's age, however. The right side of her cerebellum — the part of the brain that co-ordinates and regulates muscular activity — is slightly smaller than normal.

In one of her most recent treatments, Lisa's whole head softened, and she began to open her eyes completely. She continues to suffer from constipation, although this is better than it was. Lisa is not yet talking.

LEARNING FROM THE CASE

Lisa survived her ordeal because she is a very strong and determined child, with a totally dedicated mother. Her growth and development continue. As the nervous system released the shock, compression and layers of stress, Lisa's behavior — which looked almost "autistic" at first — improved. Her ability to communicate is developing, and she is more able to relate to others and show signs of trust. The young brain is very "plastic," and unless there is overwhelming evidence of irreparable damage, much can be done to help its development.

There are still a number of unanswered questions in Lisa's case. Was there something that could have been done sooner during Sandra's labor? Was the routine aspiration of Lisa's lungs done by someone with sufficient experience? Over the years, Lisa's parents' focus has been to organize as much collaboration as possible within the family and between all her teachers and caregivers.

The aim of Lisa's story here is to show how the concept of shock and compression being retained not only in the musculoskeletal system but also in brain tissue is a living reality. If this is not released and the normal movement of the primary respiratory mechanism restored, the self-healing ability of the body cannot function as it should. The body will then not be able to grow and develop as fully as intended.

CASE SEVEN

Rose, aged sixty-eight, was a rather extraordinary woman. She had a very rare form of cancer, which had been diagnosed when she returned to England from a vacation in Africa five years before coming to see us. The tumor was a small-cell carcinoma that was leaking serotonin (a hormone) and was in her right lung. Rose had her right lung removed, followed by radiation therapy. As a complication, she suffered from pneumonia and was expected to live only a few months.

A year later, medical investigations revealed further tumors in the muscle of her heart and in the center of her chest. Rose then had a second operation, followed by radiotherapy for over a year. This treatment scarred the lower two thirds of her esophagus and blocked the superior vena cava (vein), which made it difficult for her to swallow dry food. The superficial veins in her chest became swollen, and Rose found breathing difficult when bending over.

Rose was under the care of a professor of clinical pharmacology, whom she usually visited every six months. One month prior to her first visit to us Rose had an MRI scan of her neck, which showed marked degenerative changes for the worse, especially in the last two intervertebral discs.

Originally Rose worked as a highly specialized researcher in the field of multiple sclerosis. In her late thirties she decided to move out of this work because of professional problems. Soon after, she enrolled as a nun in a contemplative order, dedicating her time to a life of prayer. She was also a painter, who loved gardening and walking. A few years previous to the diagnosis of cancer, Rose became a Mother Superior.

THE FIRST VISIT

On her first visit to us, Rose complained of a pain in her head that travelled from the bottom of the back of her head, behind the right ear, up to the right nostril, spreading sometimes to the right side of her jaw. She had been suffering with this pain for the past twelve months. It was worse when she was lying down, and during the night she woke up every hour feeling sick. Rose also complained of a "bone pain" in her upper and lower neck, which she described as a gnawing ache. There was a grinding sound in the joints when she turned her head.

Rose found it impossible to take anti-inflammatory drugs and pain killers because they made her nauseous.

THE EXAMINATION

Rose was very calm, gentle and direct, usually smiling even while suffering the most varied combination of symptoms and what may have been considerable pain.

On examination we found a large scar on the front of her chest where the operations had been performed. She was generally tense between the neck and the abdomen, with restrictions in her spine at the level of the upper dorsal vertebrae. Both trapezeii (see the Glossary) were contracted. The movement in her neck was confused, in that when it was turned for her in one direction, the small muscles pulled it in a different one. Her neck muscles were tense.

The primary respiratory mechanism was present, but stronger in the lower half of her body; it was particularly lacking in the back of her head and the upper dorsal spine.

TREATMENT

Rose had treatment at two-week intervals for over fifteen months, dealing with a wide range of differing symptoms. At each session a specific problem would present itself for us to deal with. Some of these problems were the direct result of the increased level of serotonin while the secondary tumors were slowly growing.

It was often difficult to understand which osteopathic lesions were influencing which symptoms. However, after each session the specific symptoms were usually resolved. It was inspiring to see how, even at that late stage in her illness, Rose responded to treatment. She remained completely aware, and used to follow all the treatments with great care, asking questions and giving feedback.

OUTCOME

After the third treatment, which released the upper neck, the pain completely vanished for two months. The pain in Rose's right eye returned from time to time, but she managed to sleep for much longer periods at a time.

Nine months later, two small tumors — which Rose named Boris and Gleb — appeared at the base of her neck on the right. These gradually grew, and increased her rate of breathing, with continual rasping and loss of voice. Because her vocal cords collapsed, the surgeon wanted to inject them with silicone, which Rose chose not to have done. Subsequently, an osteopathic treatment was given to release the tension in her neck, directly working on the tumors and the surrounding fascia. During this session Rose's breathing became normal again, and her voice returned. This effect lasted for a couple of weeks before the symptoms came back, by which time Rose was needing oxygen, especially when she awoke during the night.

It was then clear that our treatment was ceasing to have lasting effects. Rose was still anxious to continue, but the benefit of treatment never lasted more than a day or so. She began a new medication for the returning and increasing bouts of nausea and was also put on low doses of morphine. However, on "good days," she was still getting up, having a meal with the sisters and taking a short walk in the garden. Three months later, in a hospice where she had gone for two weeks' respite care, on one of her good days, Rose died.

LEARNING FROM THE CASE

Rose's story illustrates that even when the body is struggling with a terminal disease, it may still benefit from osteopathic treatment. It also testifies to the tremendous courage and faith of Rose, who was one of the "sanest" people we have ever met. She had within her a feeling of being blessed, which emanated despite her suffering. She was in a state of "health" that was beyond the limitations of the body. With her life, she taught those around her that even when dying from a terminal illness you can die completely "healed."

It is arguable that Rose's illness was partly the result of somatization and the internalizing of the stress she was under in her highly responsible and "giving" position as Mother Superior. There were certainly enormous changes in the community in which she lived at that time. However, the presence of her serenity, acceptance and openness was in itself a reality.

It is possible to see people healing themselves from terminal diseases through a radical transformation of their lives and the development of a new and deep conscious awareness. Some others will instead die of their disease, but the illness itself can be in some way an integral part of their healing process.

CASE EIGHT

Stanley, aged fifty-four and a former sales manager for an advertising company, came to us complaining of a persistent and continuous pain in the back of his head on the left, spreading over to the left eye. He sometimes felt the pain inside the eye, with stiffness in the left side of his neck. It was a dull, throbbing and constant ache that was not relieved or made worse by anything. The sight in Stanley's left eye had deteriorated in the last six months.

Stanley's problems began when he was forty-six. While out walking with his wife, he became suddenly disorientated and fainted. When he came around, he had a numbness in his left side and a weakness that lasted several hours. Both before and after the incident he had a headache. Over the next three years these attacks gradually got worse until Stanley was getting them three times a week and was forced to give up his job — in itself very stressful for him. He stayed at home, afraid to go out, and completely dependent on his wife.

Three brain scans in seven years showed no abnormalities. Stanley also took an anti-epileptic drug for six months, which did not help. After seven years he had behavioral therapy from a psychotherapist for six months during which time the attacks stopped. The aim of this therapy was to help Stanley to overcome his fear and regain his confidence and independence by decreasing his anxiety. He was encouraged to do things alone and to take up some of his old interests. He was also given advice on his diet, urged to take regular exercise and taught relaxation.

Despite this therapy, though, the headaches — which had become constant — continued. After trying injections and freezing of the nerve, both of which failed to give lasting relief, Stanley was advised to have surgery. His behavioral therapist recommended a course of osteopathic treatments.

Stanley was a tall man, moderately well built, who appeared anxious and did not talk fluently. He had been unemployed for the last five years but did odd jobs in a residential home for the elderly. He drank six cups of coffee a day. At the age of twenty-one he suffered from a duodenal ulcer, and between thirty-seven and forty-seven he was on medication for high blood pressure. At that time he weighed two hundred twenty-four pounds; having lost forty-two pounds he was able to stop taking the medication. However, no improvement began in the frequency and severity of the attacks until a year later.

THE EXAMINATION

Stanley had poor muscle tone generally throughout his body. There were strong restrictions in the upper cervical spine, which was tender to the touch, especially on the left. An inflamed nodule was present in this area where Stanley had been given injections. His spine was particularly restricted where the neck joins the upper dorsal spine and at the junction between the dorsal and lumbar vertebrae. The fascia pulled his shoulders toward the upper part of his neck and the back of his head.

The primary respiratory mechanism revealed a compression in the center of Stanley's head and in the parietal bones. His membrane system was particularly tight. The examination also revealed an area of increased sensitivity to pain and touch on the skin over his left forehead, a sign that a branch of the trigeminal nerve was involved (see the Glossary).

A number of questions emerged from our osteopathic examination of Stanley and from his case history:

- Which parts of his structure are not moving normally?
- How can this influence his function and symptoms?
- Where is his circulation poor?
- What other factors can we see that may be influencing his immediate problem?
- What is the chronological order of symptoms in his life and what are the possible effects on him?
- Is Stanley a suitable case for osteopathic treatment? (In other words, does he have a significant musculoskeletal dysfunction that can be related to his problem?)

STRESS AS A CAUSE OF STANLEY'S PROBLEM

Looking at Stanley's medical history, it is clear that he suffered an autonomic nervous system (see the Glossary) imbalance for years and that stress was the common underlying factor in all his symptoms — a duodenal ulcer, obesity, poor diet, high blood pressure and headaches/attacks.

The autonomic nervous system works as a mediator between the musculoskeletal system and the viscera. It is linked to the emotional centers of the brain. It is responsible for the healthy workings of the duodenum and it also regulates the blood pressure.

Stanley is someone who easily absorbs the stresses of life into his body — known as somatization. The stress response is a natural response to situations that create fear, shock, trauma and infection. The "fight or flight" impulse in the body increases the levels of adrenaline, which causes a flow of blood toward the muscles and the brain, the heart to beat faster, the eyes to dilate and the digestion to stop. Adrenaline is not normally present in the blood — but may be in those individuals who have been under stress for years.

Prolonged stress can create biochemical changes in the body, which may interfere with normal physiological and psychological function, reducing the body's ability to respond to additional stress when it arises. Some people learn to be aware of stress without taking it onboard or allowing it to disrupt their lives.

In modern life we are exposed to continuous stress in the form of pollution, increased social chaos, time pressures, financial insecurity and emotional instability. In the late twentieth century we are in danger of losing touch with ourselves. We are in the "age of information," and so a lot of our time and energy is spent in the most superficial aspect of our minds, with little awareness of conscious physical and intellectual activity. To be in touch means to experience life in its totality with an open, feeling, thinking mind — in a conscious way that allows a free, clear and dynamic connection between the mind and the body.

We do not know what stress Stanley experienced in his life, but we know that he was greatly helped by a therapist. So it seems reasonable to assume that some of his problems at least were psychological. However, actual structural changes were clear in his body, and these may also have been a somatic response to years of excessive tension. Emotions, feelings and thoughts are all reflected in the body, which reacts to them by changes in posture and by altering its cellular make-up. Some of the changes that took place in Stanley's body persisted even after he had resolved some of the stresses involved in the lesion pattern revealed in his osteopathic examination.

In all types of pain, fear is a major factor. Chronic pain is usually associated with a negative attitude over a long period of time, and/or an unconscious emotional block. This keeps a person continually in a state of stress and so unexpressed thoughts, emotions and feelings may become locked in the body as trapped energy.

TREATMENT

Stanley had weekly treatments over a period of three months. Direct techniques were used to release the restrictions in the spine, after specific adjusting technique; the contracted fascia was unwound and the compressions in his head resolved. At one point during the treatment Stanley had a recurrence of the lower back pain he had suffered from years before, which was locally treated.

Stanley was given exercises and advice on relaxation. We also recommended that he stop drinking coffee.

OUTCOME

Stanley felt an immediate relief after the first treatment and his headache disappeared for two days. It then returned, however, and it was not until the third month that some lasting changes occurred.

As the treatment progressed, Stanley's personality began to change and he became more confident. He talked more freely, applied for a new job, and reached the point of being almost totally free of pain, with only the occasional weekend tension headache.

Stanley's story shows how an osteopath thinks when looking at a patient and his series of problems. It also shows how the whole body is interconnected — mind-matter-motion — and how trained, skilled hands can help resolve even persistent problems.

It often takes courage on the part of the patient to face themselves and to look at their problem areas. The process of healing depends on many factors, including the vitality of the patient, how precise the diagnosis and treatment procedures are, as well as the depth of communication between the practitioner and the patient. To let go and grow requires a certain state of vulnerability, which you can feel if there is trust and willingness on both sides.

RESOURCES

American Osteopathic Association (AOA)
142 East Ontario Street
Chicago, IL 60611-2864
Tel.: 312 280 5800

American Academy of Osteopathy (AAO)
3500 DePauw Boulevard, Suite 1080
Indianapolis, IN 46268-1136
Tel.: 317 879 1881

Cranial Academy (CA)
8606 Allisonville Road, Suite 130
Indianapolis, IN 46250-1136
Tel.: 317 549 0411

Sutherland Cranial Teaching Foundation (SCTF)
4116 Hartwood Drive
Fort Worth, TX 76109
Tel.: 817 735 2498

Osteopathic Center for Children (OCC)
4135 54th Place
San Diego, CA 92105
Tel.: 619 583 7611

Canadian Osteopathic Association (COA)
575 Waterloo Street
London, Ontario N6B 2R2
Tel.: 519 439 5521

RECOMMENDED READING

Anderson, Bob, *Stretching*, London: Penguin 1981.

Balaskas, Janet and Gordon, Yehudi, *The Encyclopedia of Pregnancy and Birth*, London: Macdonald 1987.

Barlow, Wilfred, *The Alexander Principle*, Essex: Anchor Brenden Ltd. 1986.

Barral, Jean Pierre, *Visceral Manipulation*, USA: Eastland Press 1993.

Blechsmidt, E., *The Beginnings of Human Life*, New York: Springer-Verlag 1977.

Chaitow, Leon, *Osteopathic Self-Treatment*, London: Thorsons 1990.

Cousins, Norman, *Anatomy of an Illness*, New York: Norton 1979.

Davidson, John, *The Web of Life*, Saffron Walden: C. W. Daniel 1988.

Dummer, Tom, *Specific Adjusting Technique*, Hove: Jotom Publications 1996.

Dummer, Tom, *Tibetan Medicine and Other Holistic Health Care Systems*, New Delhi: Paljor Publications 1995.

Feely, Richard A., *Clinical Cranial Osteopathy*, USA: Cranial Academy 1988.

Frymann, Viola, *The Cranial Letter*, (Vol. 48) USA: Cranial Academy 1995.

GCRO, *Competences Required for Osteopathic Practice*, Reading: General Council and Register of Osteopaths 1993.

Hall,T. E., and Wernham, J., *The Contribution of JML to Osteopathy*, UK: Maidstone Osteopathic Clinic 1974.

Handoll, Nicholas, *Osteopathy in Britain*, London: Osteopathic Supplies 1986.

Hartman, Laurie, *Osteopathic Technique*, London: British School of Osteopathy 1983.

Hildreth, Arthur Grant, *The Lengthening Shadow of Dr. A. T. Still*, USA: Mrs. A. G. Hildreth 1942.

Hoag, Coal and Bradford, *Osteopathic Medicine*, USA: McGraw Hill 1969.

Holmes, Pamela, "Cranial Osteopathy," in *Nursing Times* (Vol. 87, No. 22).

Isaacson, Cheryl, "Are You a Head Case?" in *Here's Health* 1985.

Korth, Stuart, "Chronic Neurological Dysfunction in Children," in *British Osteopathic Journal* (Vol. XV, 1995).

Kubler-Ross, Elisabeth, *Questions and Answers on Death and Dying*, New York: Macmillan 1974.

Latey, Dr. Philip, "Osteopathy Ancient and Modern — Still and Osteopathy Before 1900" in *Australian Journal of Osteopathy* (1990 and 1991).

Masters, Paul, *Osteopathy for Everyone*, London: Penguin 1988.

Maturana, H. R. and Varela, F. J., *Autopeosis and Cognition: The Realisation of Living*, Holland: D. Reidel 1980.

Maturana, H. R. and Varela, F. J., *The Tree of Knowledge*, USA: Shambhala 1987.

Mitchell, F. L., *Manual of Osteopathic Muscle Energy Procedures*, USA: Mitchell, Oran and Pruzzo 1979.

Pascoe, Martin, "Cranial Osteopathy," in *Nursing Times* May 1991.

Peterson, Barbara (Ed.), "On Osteopathy and Evolution," in *The Collected Papers of Irvin Korr*, USA: American Academy 1979.

Siegel, Bernie, *Love, Medicine and Miracles*, London: Rider 1986.

Skynner, Robin and Cleese, John, *Families and How to Survive Them*, London: Methuen 1984.

Smith, Fritz Frederick, *Inner Bridges*, USA: Humanics 1986.

Still, Andrew Taylor, *The Philosophy and Mechanical Principles of Osteopathy*, USA: Hudson Kimberley 1902.

Sutherland, Adah Strand, *With Thinking Fingers*, USA: Cranial Academy 1962.

Swan, Keith (Ed.), *Journal of the Osteopathic Cranial Association*, (Vol. 3, May 1991).

Todd, Mabel E., *The Thinking Body*, USA: Princeton 1949.

Trowbridge, Carol, *Andrew Taylor Still: 1828–1917*, USA: Thomas Jefferson University Press 1991.

Turner, Susan, "The Beginning — Osteopathic Care for Children," in *Journal of Osteopathic Education* (Vol. 4, Lecture Notes).

Tyreman, Stephen, "The Concepts of Disease and Health," in *Journal of Osteopathic Education* (Vol. 4, No. 1).

GLOSSARY

___

Some of the following definitions are osteopathic and differ from medical terms.

Alexander Technique: A method of posture training based on the principle that use affects function. Pioneered by Matthias Alexander (1870-1957).

Apgar score: A number from 1 to 10 given to newborn infants immediately after birth to indicate their condition.

Appendicular joints: Relating to the limbs (as opposed to axial, which refers to the trunk of the body).

Autonomic nervous system: The part of the nervous system that is involuntary, or automatic, and is concerned with regulating the activity of cardiac and smooth muscles and glands.

Bind: The point we feel when we are up against resistance while moving a structure.

Biological cognition: As a biological process, cognition is the ability of a system to modify itself in order to stay alive. Homeostasis (see below) is the result of the biological cognitive process.

Bronchus: Windpipe. Any of the larger air passages of the lungs.

Cervical spine: Part of the vertebral column formed by seven vertebrae that can be referred to by a capital letter C followed by a number, which indicates its position in the column. C1 is the one immediately underneath the back of the head (the occiput); C7 is found at the point of attachment of the neck with the shoulders.

Chiropractic: A system of therapeutics based upon the claim that disease is caused by the abnormal functioning of the nervous system. It is a manual therapy.

Cortical: Relating to the outer layer of an organ or other structure of the body, as opposed to the internal matter.

Cranial osteopathy: See Chapter Six, "The Primary Respiratory Mechanism."

Dorsal spine: Part of the vertebral column formed by twelve vertebrae found between the cervical and lumbar spine. May be referred to by using the capital letter D, followed by a number, which indicates its position in the column. The ribs are attached to each dorsal vertebra, so the dorsal spine is the backbone of the thoracic cage.

Dyslexia: Difficulty in reading and writing that bears no relation to a person's intelligence.

Ease: Ease of movement felt by palpating fingers when an action is begun.

Eclectic: Having ideas, opinions, tastes, etc., from different systems, especially in philosophy.

Endocrine system: A collection of glands that produce chemical messengers or hormones.

Excursion: Any movement from one point to another, usually with the intention of returning to the original position.

Facilitation: The state in which the nervous system can respond more quickly and easily to nervous impulses due to a lower threshold of sensory and motor reflexes.

Fascia: A sheet or band of fibrous, slightly elastic tissue that lies under the skin, and deep inside the body, enclosing the muscles, bones and all the organs. Its function is a supportive and connective one and it carries the nerves and blood vessels.

Homeopathy: A system of treatment in which diseases are treated by minute doses of drugs that in a healthy person can create symptoms like those of the disease to be treated — the principle of "like cures like." Founded by Samuel Hahnemann (1755–1843).

Homeostasis: The physiological tendency of the body to maintain the function of each of its systems within preset limits and to rebalance them when they become disrupted.

Ilium(a): Broad, flaring bone that makes up the side of the pelvis.

Immune system: The body's defense mechanism.

Interneuron: Any neuron in a chain of neurons that is situated between a sensory neuron and the final motor neuron (see Neuron).

Involuntary nervous system: See autonomic nervous system.

Ligament: A band of fibrous tissue that connects bones or cartilages, serving to strengthen and support joints.

Lymph: A transparent, slightly yellow liquid, found in the lymphatic system, which drains and cleans body tissues.

Lumbar spine: Lower end of the vertebral column. Consists of five vertebrae from the lower dorsal vertebra to the sacrum. They are referred to by using the capital letter L followed by a number from 1 to 5. The fifth is the lowest and closest to the sacrum (found between the hip bones of the pelvis).

Magnetic healing: See Mesmerism.

Malocclusion: Sufficiently poor positioning and contact between the teeth as to interfere with the movement of the jaw during chewing.

Mandible: A bone of the lower jaw.

Maxilla(e): A bone of the upper jaw.

Meconium: A dark green, sticky substance found in the intestine of the full-term fetus. It is a mixture of secretions from the intestinal glands and some amniotic fluid.

Mediastinum: The mass of tissues and organs separating the two lungs, between the sternum (breastbone) and the vertebral column.

Mesmerism: Introduced in 1836 and popularly known as magnetic healing. Practitioners believed that there was an invisible fluid—called animal magnetism—flowing through the body, which when equally balanced meant good health. Mesmerism attempts to restore balance through rubbing, will power, concentration and sometimes techniques similar to those used in exorcism. It was later adapted into hypnotism.

Mobility: Free movement between body structures.

Motility: Movement within every structure.

Muscle chain: A group of muscles that are linked in a functional chain.

Neuron: Nervous system cell, which transmits impulses.

Occiput: The bone at the back of the head.

Osteopathic inhibition: See Chapter Five, "Osteopathic Techniques."

Osteopathic lesion (or Somatic dysfunction): See Chapter Three, "The Osteopathic Lesion."

Osteophyte: A bony outgrowth.

Osteoporosis: Reduction in the density of bone, resulting in brittle and fragile bones. Especially common in women after menopause.

Palatal: Relating to the palate.

Palpation: Manual means of diagnosing a problem whereby sensory information is received through the fingers and hands.

Parasympathetic nervous system: Part of the autonomic nervous system with nerves arising from the cranium (skull) and sacrum.

Parietal bone: A bone of the cranium (skull).

Pathology: This is a medical term, defined as the essential nature of disease.

Peridontal: Relating to the tissues or region around a tooth.

Perinatal: The period between the seventh month of pregnancy and the first week of life.

Pharmacology: The science of drugs.

Phrenology: A science of natural law, established in the 1850s. It claimed that the body was part of the universe and governed by universal laws. By following these laws the health and mind of the individual could be improved. Phrenologists offered character analysis by reading the bumps on a person's cranium.

Physiology: The scientific study of living things and their parts.

Physiotherapy: The treatment of disease and injury by methods including manipulation, massage and remedial exercise, without drugs.

Primary respiratory mechanism (PRM): See Chapter Six.

Proprioceptive: The special function of sensory nerve end organs found in muscles, tendons and joints, whereby they monitor the position of the muscle, etc., in space or posture.

Psoas: Lower back muscles that insert on the lumbar vertebrae and discs, pass through the pelvis and insert on the inner part of the femur (thigh-bone).

Sacrum: A triangular shaped bone made from fused vertebrae, and found between the two hip bones of the pelvis.

Solar plexus: Situated between the diaphragm and the umbilicus (navel), this is a bundle of radiating nerves.

Somatic: Body structures (as opposed to those of the mind).

Somatic dysfunction (or Osteopathic lesion): See Chapter Three, "The Osteopathic Lesion."

Spasticity: An increase in the normal tone of a muscle due to the presence of a pathology.

Sphenoid bone: Irregular, butterfly-shaped bone in the skull, behind the eyes.

Spiritualism: A belief that the spirits of the dead can communicate with the living world through sensitive people such as mediums.

Sympathetic nervous system: Part of the autonomic nervous system that arises from the spinal cord in the thoracic and lumbar regions.

Temporal: Bone in the cranium found under the outside part of the ear.

Temporomandibular joint: Where the jaw bone meets the cranium at the temporal bone.

Tendon: A cord, band or sheet or fibrous tissue attaching a muscle to a bone or other structure.

Torcicollis: When the cervical muscles are contracted, producing twisting of the neck and an unnatural position of the head.

Torsion: The condition of being twisted.

Toxicity: In osteopathy, tissues can be referred to as having a toxic quality. This may be caused by poor diet, poor metabolism, drugs that have not been eliminated from the body, allergy or areas of inactivity.

Tracheotomy: A small cut on the front of the throat to put a tube into the windpipe to assist air-flow.

Trapezius: A large muscle that covers the upper back, spanning from the occiput (see above) to the twelfth dorsal vertebra and across to both shoulders.

Trigeminal nerve: The fifth cranial nerve supplying the face and the chewing muscles.

Vascular: Relating to blood vessels.

Ventouse extraction: A means of delivering a baby where a suction cap is attached to the baby's scalp and the baby is pulled out.

Ventral: Same as anterior in human anatomy.

Vertebra: One of the bony units of the vertebral column.

Visceral: Relating to any large internal organ in any of the three great cavities of the body.

Visceral technique: Osteopathic technique developed mainly for the manipulation of an internal organ. See Chapter Five, "Osteopathic Techniques."

Zygoma: A bone in the face that forms part of the orbit.

INDEX

NOTES

NOTES

NOTES

NOTES

NOTES

NOTES

OTHER ULYSSES PRESS
HEALTH TITLES

ANXIETY AND DEPRESSION: A NATURAL APPROACH
Shirley Trickett

By addressing the patient's total health from a physical *and* mental standpoint, *Anxiety and Depression: A Natural Approach* avoids the failure of traditional medical treatment. With specific suggestions on diet, breathing, relaxation, bio-feedback, and exercise, the program helps sufferers empower themselves to prevent further discomfort. $8.95

THE BOOK OF KOMBUCHA
Beth Ann Petro

The Book of Kombucha explains the health benefits of the "tea mushroom" while answering the concerns surrounding this alternative health treatment. Draws on up-to-date research and explains how to grow and use Kombucha. $11.95

BREAKING THE AGE BARRIER:
STAYING YOUNG, HEALTHY AND VIBRANT
Helen Franks

Drawing on the latest medical research, *Breaking the Age Barrier* explains how the proper lifestyle can stop the aging process and make you feel youthful and vital. $12.95

COUNT OUT CHOLESTEROL
Art Ulene, M.D. and Val Ulene, M.D.

Complete with counter and detailed dietary plan, this companion resource to the *Count Out Cholesterol Cookbook* shows how to design a cholesterol-lowering program that's right for you. $12.95

COUNT OUT CHOLESTEROL COOKBOOK
Art Ulene, M.D. and Val Ulene, M.D.

A companion guide to *Count Out Cholesterol*, this book shows you how to bring your cholesterol levels down with the help of 250 gourmet recipes. $14.95

DISCOVER MEDITATION: A FIRST-STEP GUIDE TO BETTER HEALTH
Doriel Hall

> *Discover Meditation* leads the reader step by step through a journey of discovery into this ancient discipline. Chapters address everything from physical positioning and breathing techniques to focusing the mind and achieving self-knowledge. $8.95

DISCOVER OSTEOPATHY: A FIRST-STEP GUIDE TO BETTER HEALTH
Peta Sneddon and Paolo Coseschi

> In *Discover Osteopathy,* two practicing osteopaths explain simply and lucidly the basic principles of osteopathy, when to visit an osteopath, and how osteopathy works. Specific chapters detail osteopathic techniques, and special sections look at the application of these therapies in areas like pregnancy, childbirth, and even dentistry. $8.95

DISCOVER REFLEXOLOGY: A FIRST-STEP GUIDE TO BETTER HEALTH
Rosalind Oxenford

> *Discover Reflexology* relates this ancient tradition to its historical context within Chinese medicine and to the modern understanding of holistic health programs that address body, mind, and spirit. This book empowers the beginner to incorporate the therapy into his or her own personal program of good health. $8.95

DISCOVERY PLAY
Art Ulene, M.D. and Steven Shelov, M.D.

> This book guides parents through the first three years of their child's life, offering play activity with a special emphasis on nurturing self-esteem. $9.95

IRRITABLE BOWEL SYNDROME: A NATURAL APPROACH
Rosemary Nicol

> This book offers a natural approach to a problem millions of sufferers have. The author clearly defines the symptoms and offers a dietary and stress-reduction program for relieving the effects of this disease. $9.95

KNOW YOUR BODY: THE ATLAS OF ANATOMY
Introduction by Trevor Weston, M.D.

> Designed to provide a comprehensive and concise guide to the structure of the human body, *Know Your Body* offers more than 250 color illustrations. An easy-to-follow road map of the human body. $12.95

LAST WISHES: A HANDBOOK TO GUIDE YOUR SURVIVORS
Lucinda Page Knox, M.S.W. and Michael D. Knox, Ph.D.

> A simple do-it-yourself workbook, *Last Wishes* helps people put their affairs in order and eases the burden on their survivors. It allows them to plan their own funeral and leave final instructions for survivors. $12.95

LOSE WEIGHT WITH DR. ART ULENE
Art Ulene, M.D.

> This best-selling weight-loss book offers a 28-day program for taking off the pounds and keeping them off forever. $12.95

MOOD FOODS
William Vayda

> *Mood Foods* shows how the foods you eat can influence your emotions, behavior, and personality. It also explains how a proper diet can help to alleviate such common complaints as PMS, hyperactivity, mood swings, and stress. $9.95

PANIC ATTACKS: A NATURAL APPROACH
Shirley Trickett

> Addresses the problem of panic attacks using a holistic approach. Focusing on diet and relaxation, the book helps you prevent future attacks. $8.95

THE VITAMIN STRATEGY
Art Ulene, M.D. and Val Ulene, M.D.

> A game plan for good health, this book helps readers design a vitamin and mineral program tailored to their individual needs. $11.95

YOUR NATURAL PREGNANCY:
A GUIDE TO COMPLEMENTARY THERAPIES
Anne Charlish

> This timely book brings together the many complementary therapies such as aromatherapy, massage, homeopathy, acupressure, herbal medicine, and meditation, that can benefit pregnant women. $16.95

To order these or other Ulysses Press books call 800-377-2542 or write to Ulysses Press, P.O. Box 3440, Berkeley, CA 94703-3440. All retail orders are shipped free of charge. California residents must include sales tax. Allow two to three weeks for delivery.

Peta Sneddon and Paolo Coseschi are registered osteopaths who share a private practice in Chianti, Italy.